TABLE OF CO

Top 20 Test Taking Tips

1. Carefully follow all the test registration procedures
2. Know the test directions, duration, topics, question types, how many questions
3. Setup a flexible study schedule at least 3-4 weeks before test day
4. Study during the time of day you are most alert, relaxed, and stress free
5. Maximize your learning style; visual learner use visual study aids, auditory learner use auditory study aids
6. Focus on your weakest knowledge base
7. Find a study partner to review with and help clarify questions
8. Practice, practice, practice
9. Get a good night's sleep; don't try to cram the night before the test
10. Eat a well balanced meal
11. Know the exact physical location of the testing site; drive the route to the site prior to test day
12. Bring a set of ear plugs; the testing center could be noisy
13. Wear comfortable, loose fitting, layered clothing to the testing center; prepare for it to be either cold or hot during the test
14. Bring at least 2 current forms of ID to the testing center
15. Arrive to the test early; be prepared to wait and be patient
16. Eliminate the obviously wrong answer choices, then guess the first remaining choice
17. Pace yourself; don't rush, but keep working and move on if you get stuck
18. Maintain a positive attitude even if the test is going poorly
19. Keep your first answer unless you are positive it is wrong
20. Check your work, don't make a careless mistake

Degenerative Disease

Osteoarthritis

Osteoarthritis is the most common of the degenerative diseases. Although, osteoarthritis may actually be developing as early as the second or third decade, it is often asymptomatic until after age 50 at which time there is also likely to be radiological evidence as well. Some literature suggests that greater than 80% of the 55-and-older population will demonstrate signs of osteoarthritis on x-ray, whether they are symptomatic or not. Osteoarthritis is diagnosed earlier in the knees of females than males and is thought to be twice that of males. Hip osteoarthritis is diagnosed equally in males and females. Other common joints involved in this process are back, hands/fingers and shoulder.

The etiology of osteoarthritis: Osteoarthritis is primarily a disease of the cartilage in between joints. The etiology of osteoarthritis is still unclear. However, there are many theories. Ostoeoarthritis is no longer simply being defined as a "wear and tear" of the joints. There are a number of factors that may contribute to the formation of this degenerative disease. Age, obesity and excessive stress on the joints from sports and certain occupations can be considered "wear and tear" and are still among the etiologies for this degenerative disease. Furthermore, single or repetitive joint injury, improperly formed joints, poorly developed muscles and genetic defect in the joint cartilage itself are other theories as to the origin of osteoarthritis.

Cartilage is made primarily of collagen, a protein. Joint cartilage is made up of two main components. These are extracellular matrix and chondrocytes, which are contained within the matrix. The extracellular matrix contains primarily type II, IX and XI collagens as well as aggrecan proteoglycans. Type II collagen is largely responsible for protecting the ends of the bone within a joint. Aggrecan proteoglycans are mainly responsible for retaining water molecules, allowing resistance to affects of strenuous use on the joint. The chondrocytes within the matrix itself are largely responsible for the strength and resistance to loading on the cartilage.

Pathology of osteoarthritis: Healthy cartilage provides a joint with minimal friction with movements. When the cartilage becomes damaged in the early stages it starts to lose its elasticity, making it more susceptible to injury. With increasing stress and wear on the overlying cartilage, the underlying bone starts to become affected. Thickening of the bone and formation of bone spurs and osteophytes, usually at the edges of the joint, can evidence this. Some of these abnormal bone formations may break loose with cartilage fragments and float within the joint space. This debris within the joint space causes the synovium to mount and inflammatory response to break down the cartilaginous debris. However, this inflammatory response also increases the breakdown of the remaining healthy cartilage, leading to further degenerative changes in the joint.

Symptoms of osteoarthritis: Patients are likely to complain of pain and stiffness. Pain is likely to be exacerbated with activity and better with rest (early disease). They may complain of swelling. Pain and stiffness may be worse in the morning (no more than 30 minutes). Pain may be worse with prolonged inactivity or with weather changes. If osteoarthritis is present in the hips, complaints may include pain in the low back and groin, limping and knee pain from compensation. Knee complaints may include locking, cracking and grinding, feeling as if the knee is going to "give out" and increasing pain with ascending and descending stairs. Finger complaints may be swelling, nodules, stiffness and difficulty gripping.

Some common causes of secondary osteoarthritis include: Joint injury- any condition causing fracture or sprain would be included in joint injury. Chronic stress- on a joint may come from an occupation that causes repetitive use or stress on a joint (landscaping, typing and athletes) or females that wears high-heeled shoes frequently. Joint instability-can put more stress on the joint from injury to surrounding soft-tissue structures of the joint such as tendon and ligament injury or poor conditioning and muscle strength. Nervous system disorders- causing secondary osteoarthritis includes: Charcot neuropathy or any disorder that affects proprioception and thus movements. Blood and endocrine disorders- that can cause secondary osteoarthritis are diabetes, gout, thyroid disorders, osteoarthritis, and growth hormone disorders. Medications- that can contribute to osteoarthritis are oral steroids and medications used to treat gout. Inflammation- in joints secondary to disorders such as rheumatoid arthritis and injuries can cause secondary osteoarthritis.

It is important to differentiate between osteoarthritis and other diseases. Nursing history should include description of pain: location, nature, frequency, intensity, exacerbating and alleviating factors, time of day, time of year (weather changes) and if pain radiates. Note patient age, gender, occupation, hobbies, injury history and family history. Determine how this affects activities of daily living and have them give examples (ascending/descending stairs, opening jars, rising from chair, writing, dressing and hygiene). Determine if it has caused them to perform tasks differently or avoid certain activities. Have their symptoms affected their job performance? Assessment and history should also include how it is affecting them emotionally; include assessing sleeping, eating and sexual activity changes. Evaluate support system. Determine previous diagnosis or diagnostic work-up.

Goals of management are to reduce pain and inflammation and maintain or increase joint function. Management and goals should be met with nonpharmacological therapy first. If pharmacological therapy is necessary, it should be with the smallest amount and for the shortest period of time needed to reduce pain and help function. Management should allow patient to maintain independence and confidence with activities of daily living. Osteoarthritis limitations should be addressed by corrective parameters of already existing disability and preventive measure to prevent further disability. Patient education, regarding the disorder and any medications or assistive devices being used, is important. The importance of maintaining range of motion, muscle strength and reducing stress on joints should be taught and demonstrated. Finally, goals should include collaboration among other health care professionals including doctors, midlevel providers, nurses, therapists, counselors, and specialists.

Diagnostic tests should be considered to confirm physical findings. Laboratory or blood tests are not mandatory for diagnosis of osteoarthritis itself; however, it is important for eliminating other similar presenting disorders such as rheumatoid arthritis. It also helps determine additional underlying disorders that may be responsible for secondary osteoarthritis such as gout or thyroid disorder. Finally, blood work is important for establishing a baseline before initiating therapy or to help determine therapy. Imaging studies are a mainstay of osteoarthritis diagnosis. X-rays are the most common and cost-effective initially; however, it is not unusual for MRI and bone scans to be utilized. Findings on x-ray may include: joint space narrowing, bone spurs and osteophytes. Evaluation of synovial fluid via joint aspiration is necessary. Synovial fluid of osteoarthritis will likely be straw colored, contain no greater than 2000 white blood cells/mm^3, and synovial glucose should be equivalent to serum glucose.

Some alternative treatments (approved and unapproved) that your osteoarthritis patients may ask you about:

Glucosamine: oral, thought to regenerate joint cartilage. There are some good studies supporting its use to reduce pain and inflammation.
SAM-e: oral, thought to reduce pain in osteoarthritis. Support and studies vary.
Copper and Magnetic bracelets: anecdotal reports only. Scientific studies do not support. No known harmful effects.
Acupuncture: many studies support benefits, others are inconclusive. Likely there is some dependence on disease progression, joint involved and acupuncturist training.
Tai Chi, Pilates, and Yoga: exercises involving slow and steady body movement, breathing and concentration.
Herbs: garlic, Echinacea, ginkgo, St. John's Wort, ginger, tumeric, and cayenne are met with varied support. The later three have more supportive studies and it is thought that their use in degenerative disease may be helpful.
Supplements: studies support Vitamin D, Vitamin C and antioxidants for their potential to stabilize degenerative disease.

There are several modifiable risk factors for the development of osteoarthritis. First and foremost in the modifiable risk category for osteoarthritis is weight. This is especially true in osteoarthritis of the back, hips and knees. This does not affect the development of osteoarthritis in non-weight bearing joints such as the hands, elbows and shoulders. Closely related to weight is the second modifiable risk factor for osteoarthritis: activity level. Regular exercise and participation in recreational activities keeps joints healthy in a number of ways: it keeps the joint surface lubricated and mobile; it helps the strength of surrounding tendons, ligaments and muscles conditioned, thus taking stress off of the joint itself; and it keeps weight down. However, excess levels of physical activity can increase the risk of wear and tear on joints and thus osteoarthritis.

There are several key points in obtaining a history of a patient with osteoarthritis. Assess pain including: location, onset/duration and type.

Assess activity including: response to, pain alleviating exacerbating activities, and fatigability. Assess effect of disorder on sleep. Assess nutritional status, unintended weight gain or loss, and note caffeine consumption. Assess activities of daily living: self-care, occupational and family roles. Assess effect on sexual relations, self-concept and image, independence, hobbies and coping mechanisms. Assess patient's support system, knowledge base of disorder, comorbidity, medications, compliance and treatments already tried. Ask about past medical history and family medical history. Note the patient's social history including use of alcohol, tobacco and drugs.

Side effects of common oral pharmacological agents

The side effects of some common oral pharmacological agents used in degenerative disease include:
Acetaminophen (Tylenol): dose should be no greater than 4000mg per day. A major side effect is liver toxicity, but this is usually only seen if the amount of acetaminophen exceeds the recommended dosage and/or more likely to be seen in patients that chronically consume large amounts of alcohol
Nonsteroidal Anti-Inflammatory drugs (NSAIDs): examples include ibuprofen and naproxyn. Serious side effects are gastric ulceration and bleed as well as renal impairment. Newer COX-2 NSAIDs such as Celebrex, significantly reduce the gastrointestinal risks.
Non-narcotic, centrally-acting analgesics: (tramadol). Side effects include vertigo, headache, nausea and constipation. Although abuse potential is significantly less than a narcotic analgesic, habituation is still possible.
Opiod (Narcotic) Analgesics: (codeine, propoxyphene). Side effects include constipation, disorientation and vertigo. Abuse potential is high. Use with caution in elderly patients. Safely added to NSAIDs, ideal use is no greater than 2 weeks at a time.

Corticosteroid injections and topical analgesics

Injection of an osteoarthritic joint is most successful in joints that demonstrate signs of inflammation and when other, more conservative, modalities have failed. Injection with a glucocorticoid can provide the patient with about three to four weeks of relief. The placebo effect of the injection is unknown, but has been questioned. It is not recommended that a single joint undergo more than three steroid injections in a single year. Topical analgesic, in combination with other treatments, has demonstrated some pain reduction. The most common and most studied is capsaicin cream, along Aspercreme, Bengay, Icy Hot, and Flexall, can be found over-the-counter. They are generally not harmful, except in cases where they are applied to a break in the skin, placed over a joint that tightly occluded. They may cause some local irritation. Compliance is an issue, because in order to get relief the cream often needs to be applied to the joint multiple times daily.

Viscosupplementation

Viscosupplementation is increasingly used in osteoarthritis of the knee. There are different formulations available. They involve a series of injections, into the knee joint, over a period of weeks. The injections are composed of hyaluronic acid, which is essentially a substance found in the human body that gives synovial fluid its thickness and cushion. Viscosupplementation is usually reserved for cases in which other treatments have failed. The goals of these injections are to improve lubrication of the joint, decrease pain and allow for increase mobility and activity. Some studies report success for up to 6 months after the injections. Viscosupplementation is not curative.

Complications after total joint replacement

Thromboembolic events such as pulmonary embolism (PE) and deep vein thrombosis (DVT) are the most common complications for total knee and hip replacement. The risk of these can be reduced by a thorough preoperative evaluation that includes: past history of social history (smoking), current medication (anticoagulants, hormones) and their preoperative cessation timing, age and other comorbidities. Preventive measures for DVT and PE are postoperative mobilization, a course of anticoagulant medication and pneumatic compression devices. Simple range of motion exercise of distal joints, especially flexion and extension, are encouraged to keep the blood flowing.

Orthopedic diagnosis example

As an example, a patient presents with the following scenario. Following the example is the most likely orthopedic diagnosis and other possible findings. Scenario: 60-year-old patient with trendelenburg and antalgic gait and inability to internally rotate at the left hip

Osteoarthritis of the left hip is the most likely diagnosis, given the patients age and findings. Of course a thorough history is important, eliminating the possibility of traumatic injury that could cause fracture or dislocation. Determine the length of time the pain has been present and the onset and progression. Check family history. Evaluate the patient for pain in the left thigh (anterior and/or lateral), left buttocks and groin, as these are common with hip osteoarthritis. There should not be defects in reflexes and muscle strength. X-rays will demonstrate decreased joint space, sclerosis and osteophyte formation.

Trendelenburg sign and gait

The trendelenburg gait and sign can be used to assess various disorders including: weakness in hip muscles, congenital defect of the hip, osteoarthritis of the hip and rheumatoid arthritis. For best results and evaluation, the top of the patient's hips and waist need to be well visualized. Have the patient remove or lift his/her shirt. It is ideal to evaluate the patient with only their underclothing on the bottom. When the patient is standing, their upper body will lean towards the affected hip and the affected hip will be lower than the non-affected hip. This is a positive trendelenburg sign. A trendelenburg gait is observed when the patient places their weight on the affected hip/leg and the opposite hip lowers. With the weight on the unaffected hip, the affected hip naturally lowers, so the alternating weight shifting involved in walking causes and exaggerated appearance of the hips rising and falling with gait.

Home exercises

Side "push-up" – lying on your left side, with knees slightly bent, hold your body up by your left elbow, keeping your body in alignment. Hold position for recommended time, and then repeat on right side. Hip thrust – lie supine with feet on the floor and knees at 90 degrees. Press small of back to the floor, hold. Now lift hips upward keeping you body (from shoulders to knees) in alignment, hold. Repeat for predetermined number of repetitions.
Knees to chest – lie supine, bend and bring left knee to chest, hold. Repeat with right knee, hold. Repeat with both knees. Crawl – get into crawl or "four-legged" position, making sure back is not arched in either direction, but flat. Extend left arm forward and in a straight line with body. At the same time, extend right leg out behind you (not to the side) and in a straight plane with your back and left arm. Hold. Repeat with opposite leg and arm.

Chronic low back pain

Lumbar pain is a common complaint. However it is important to determine if it is chronic or acute. It is also important to determine the origin and make sure it is not a result of a referred pain from other locations such as the abdomen or pelvis. A classic finding in chronic low back pain is the complaint that pain radiates to the buttocks, either unilateral or bilateral. Pain is usually exacerbated by movement of that area such as forward flexion and circumflexion at the waist, squatting, lifting or any combination of these. Alleviators are rest in the supine position. Patient will likely be tender to moderate to deep palpation at the lumbar and/or sacroiliac level. Reflexes and strength versus resistance testing should be within normal limit, if not, consider neurological origin. X-rays will likely show decreased disc space between vertebrae and osteophyte formation.

Appropriate gait

With hip osteoarthritis or after a total hip replacement, a patient may need a cane. The cane should be used on the opposite side of the affected hip, in this case the cane would be held in the right hand. After fitting patient with the appropriate cane type and height, gait review is necessary. The patient should advance the cane forward with his right hand/arm as his left leg (affected hip side) steps forward. It is important to lift the cane completely off the ground when advancing it forward, to reduce the risk of falls and to achieve maximum benefit. The left foot should land on the surface at approximately the same time as the cane in the right hand. The cane is to be used much like an "extra extremity", taking the burden off the affected/healing limb. Stairs should be the same: lead with the right leg then bring the left leg and cane up/down to the step that the right foot is already on.

Knee pain stretches

Straight-Leg Raise (stretch). While lying supine, prop yourself up on your elbows. Bend your left knee to 90 degrees with foot flat on the floor. With right leg straight, dorsiflex foot, tighten thigh muscles and lift straightened right leg off the floor about 5-10 inches, hold. Repeat with opposite leg. Lunges (strengthen). Stand with feet about 4 feet apart. Lunge forward (bend left knee) with left knee, keeping back and right leg straight. Right foot may point slightly outward to help with balance. Hands may rest on thighs, but should not bare-weight on them. Lunge forward until slight stretch is felt in the left groin, hold. Repeat with opposite leg.

Intraoperative and/or postoperative complications

Modifiable factors placing one at increased risk for surgical complications include: smoking, obesity, malnutrition, health and conditioning prior to surgery, and not discontinuing medications and the recommended interval prior to surgery. Several comorbidities also place a patient at higher risk for operative complications, including: diabetes, coronary artery disease, poorly controlled hypertension, congestive heart failure, chronic obstructive pulmonary disease, asthma, and autoimmune disease. A previous poor surgical outcome places a patient at increased risk for operative complications. Active and recurrent infection increases operative risk. Bleeding disorders, certain medications, old age and any immunocompromised condition carries an increase risk for complications. Trauma surgery places one at increased risk of surgical and post surgical complications versus elective surgery.

Abductor pillows

An abductor pillow also known as an abductor wedge or just "wedge" is used in the total hip replacement postoperative period. Its continued and chronic use is highly recommended. The wedge pillow is designed to fit between the patient's legs. This keeps the patients hips in extension, the legs in abduction and in slight external rotation. The wedge is usually strapped in place with two, slightly flexible, wide Velcro-like straps. These straps are placed approximately at the level of the lower thigh (a few inches above the knees) and the middle to lower calf. Care must be taken not to have the straps impinge upon the peroneal nerve. This nerve is present a few inches distal and lateral to the knee, and then branches distally.

Alternative therapies

Some alternative therapies for chronic degenerative back pain include the following:

Spinal manipulation, whether it be osteopathic or chiropractic, has been an approved therapy modality in some cases. It has shown the most success with newer pain versus pain that has been present for several months. Manipulation is not recommended if there are radicular symptoms or signs of neurologic deficit or compression. Furthermore, it is recommended that treatments cease if symptomology is increased or lack of improvement after one month. The TENS unit (transcutaneous electric nerve stimulation) is widely used with various results. Other possibilities work a try and with limited data are acupuncture, biofeedback and the various message techniques and sub-specialties.

Self-care recommendations

Regular stretching and exercise is important for both acute and chronic pain episodes. It is important not to prescribe 'bed rest' even for a few days, in a person with an acute exacerbation of chronic back pain. Rest weakens the muscles in the back, which are our main structural and postural muscles. Therefore, encourage movement, as this will keep muscles loose, joints lubricated and blood flowing to the injured area. Light stretching and range of motion exercises can be done immediately, slowly adding in light to non-weight bearing exercises (swimming and bicycling) to build endurance and strength. Repetitive lifting, bending and twisting are not recommended. If an activity causes pain or makes existing pain worse: stop or alter that activity. Ice is recommended for the first 48-72 hours of acute pain, beyond that, heat usually feels better and is more helpful. Review ergonomics with respect to patient's occupation/hobbies.

Surgical positioning and postoperative hip precautions

Hip replacement with anterior approach requires patient to be lying supine, hip extended and in external rotation, and knee flexed. However, anterior approach can still be accomplished with the patient in the position for the posterior approach. For posterior approach, patient lies on their unaffected side, with affected hip in flexion, adduction and internal rotation. Post-surgical hip precautions for anterior approach include: no external rotation of knees/ankles, no turning towards operative side with walking, no abduction of surgical hip and no crossing legs (ankle on knee or knee on knee). Precautions for post-surgical hip after posterior approach: no bending at the waist greater than 90 degrees, do not sit cross-legged, no internal rotation on surgical side. Posterior approach recommends sleeping with pillow between knees and external rotation of legs.

Surgical positions

The surgical positions for patients following different types of procedures are:

- Thoracic spine surgery: prone position, this position is also used with lumbar spine procedures. Elbows should be slightly flexed and be alert to pressure spots on the face.

- Total hip replacement: lateral position, affected hip up, bottom knee slightly flexed and bottom shoulder with forward flexion. Position neck so it is aligned with spine.
- Total knee replacement: supine position, with headrest to align cervical spine in comfortable and natural position, arms usually to the side.
- Open hip reduction: supine position.
- Shoulder replacement: supine, reclined position with head secured.
- Knee scope: supine with foot of bed (starting at the knee level) lowered.
- Shoulder scope: lateral position.

Chronic rotator cuff tear

Osteoarthritis of the shoulder is often caused by chronic rotator cuff tear. This is usually gradual in onset, as most degenerative disease is. Morning stiffness is common, often put off by the patient as, "I slept wrong". Over time, incidence and severity of pain increases. Eventually, the pain can actually awake the patient from sleep, if they turn wrong and apply pressure to the affected shoulder joint. Activities of daily living become more challenging and cause more pain, especially 'over head' activities that have the shoulder in greater than 90 degrees of abduction.

CPM machines

CPM machines, or continuous passive motion machines, can be used in the early postoperative period of total knee replacement, usually starting within the first 24 hours. It is a machine that the operative knee/leg is placed in to reduce stiffness and aide in the return of range of motion. It can be set to take the knee through gradual and various degrees of flexion and extension. If the patient resists this passive range of motion, the flexion-extension cycle is halted. For maximum benefit, the CPM machine should be applied at least six hours in a 24-hour period. Increases in length and degrees of range of motion are dictated by the surgeon and patient response.

Chondromalacia patellae

Of all of the degenerative disorders, this is one that can be seen in a younger age group. Also known as patellofemoral syndrome, chondromalacia patellae is a disorder where the underside or backside of the kneecap is roughened. This surface does have joint cartilage, as it comes in contact with the femur. When this joint space decreases or is no longer smooth, it causes pain with all movement that causes the kneecap to move over the femur. This can be caused from heavy use of this joint, such as a marathon runner may sustain. Trauma and poorly developed thigh muscles or quads can contribute to this disorder.

Shoulder fusion candidates

If a patient with shoulder osteoarthritis has failed at conservative treatment (non-steroidal anti-inflammatory drugs, analgesics, joint injections, and physical therapy) and shoulder pain and loss of range of motion persists, they become a candidate for surgical treatment. Shoulder fusion is one surgical option. This is a good option for a younger patient (<40) that uses their shoulder a great deal for labor-intensive occupations or participation in sports or hobbies that require a lot of upper extremity use. Shoulder fusion can be done even in a severely damaged rotator cuff. It is also the best choice for a patient that may be non-compliant in the post surgical rehabilitation program.

Bunions

Bunions are also known as hallux valgus, lateral deviation of the MTP (metatarsal phalangeal) joint of the great toe. The MTP joint degenerates over time, usually due to poorly fitting footwear. Women wearing narrow, tight-fitting and heeled shoes are an example. This may be why this is a much more common finding in females. Occasionally this will be found in younger patients as a birth anomaly. Pain is because of prominence of distal 1st metatarsal head and its susceptibility to pressure. Treatment is conservative: wider fitting shoes, shoe inserts, anti-inflammatory and analgesic medication, and injections. Surgery is only an option if the 2nd – 5th toes become affected and outward pointing and pain persists.

Crutches

Proper fitting of crutches are important to avoid nerve damage that can be sustained from too much pressure and weight bearing in the armpit, impinging upon the brachial plexus. This can also cause disruption in blood flow. Furthermore, handgrip position is important for the same reasons. With patient standing, place tip of crutch a hand length in front of and to the lateral side of the fifth toe. From here, the space between the armpit and the top of crutch should be 2 inches. Handgrip should then be adjusted with wrist in neutral position and elbow at about 30 degrees of flexion. This usually places handgrips at hip level.

There are 5 common ways to walk with crutches:

- Swing-Through: most common. Simultaneously move both crutches forward. Swing both feet forward, landing beyond the crutches. At least 2 points of contacts at all times.
- Swing-To: Both crutches moved forward, then simultaneously move both feet forward, even with crutches. Maintains minimum of 2 points of contact at all times.

- Single Swing-Through: Both crutches moved forward. Body weight is shifted to move strong leg (unaffected leg) forward beyond crutches. 2 points of contact alternate with 1 contact point.
- Four-Point: Move right crutch forward, then left foot even with right crutch. Move left crutch forward, and then right foot forward, even with left crutch. At least 3 points of contact are maintained at all times.
- Two-Point Alternating: Simultaneously move right crutch and left foot forward, and then simultaneously bring left crutch and right leg forward. 2 contact points alternate with 4.

Assistive devices

Patients with degenerative joint disease might use several different types of assistive devices. What device the patient chooses often depends on the location where it will be used.

In the bathroom: safety bars around toilets and in showers, elevated toilet seats, rubber mats in the shower to prevent slipping, long-handled sponge, rugs with no-skid backing, and shower/bath chairs can be helpful. For dressing: zipper-pull and button assisting devices. Elastic shoelaces may allow for easier on and off of shoes, without having to bend to tie them. Shoehorns of all lengths are available for helping don footwear. A variety of graspers, pinchers and reachers can be used for many things including pulling up socks and picking things up from the floor. In the kitchen: grippers and lid and can openers. Foam and gel grips are recommended for eating, cooking, and writing utensils. Work space: Seat extenders to elevate chair seats, even chair-lifts are available, movable tables that fit over bed or chair, and arm rest attachments for comfortable and ergonomic working environment.

Low back pain diagnosis

From a thorough history and physical exam, you should be able to determine if any diagnostic tests are needed. The majority of cases do not require imaging studies or labs. The few exceptions to this rule are if the low back pain was caused by traumatic injury, there is loss of bowel and bladder control, or there are signs of severe nerve damage. If these conditions are absent, a 7-10 day trial of conservative therapy can be initiated. Approximately 85% of low back pain improves with conservative measures. The patient should follow up after the period of conservative treatment, to assess its affect.

Types of pain

Different disorders and diseases cause patients to complain about pain in different ways. Some examples:

- Spondylolisthesis: Pain is usually made worse with movements at the waist such as forward flexion and circumflexion. Lifting, especially if using poor technique, can also aggravate this condition. Pain also may radiate down one leg. In more extreme cases, there may be complaints of bowel and bladder changes and decreased distal sensation.
- Herniated disc: Pain may be sudden in onset, with little or no trauma. Pain radiates to leg and is worse with sitting, bending forward, and sneezing. Sensory changes and muscular strength in the extremity may be affected.
- Spinal stenosis: Pain is aggravated when back is straight or extended, when lying supine, and can often radiate into both legs. Pain is also worse with walking, slightly relieved when hunched forward.

Conservative therapy

Conservative therapy for the patient with low back pain usually includes nonsteroidal anti-inflammatory medication, muscle relaxer medication, and narcotic or non-narcotic analgesics in some combination. Furthermore, it includes activity restrictions, but not out-right bed rest. Activity restrictions are often: no heavy or repetitive lifting, to twisting, no bending at the waist and avoidance of vibratory activities or any activity that exacerbates the pain. Instructing the patient in proper body mechanics is equally important. Ice, heat, massage, stretching and topical creams may all be recommended in various combinations. Physical therapy can be initiated at this stage or at the follow up visit. Alternative therapies may be recommended on a case-by-case basis, and are usually reserved for failure of conservative measures.

Follow-up visits

For a patient treated with conservative therapy for low back pain, a follow-up visit will include a thorough history and physical examination. This is compared to the initial visit to assess improvement or lack there of as well as to determine which conservative measures were successful. If there is improvement, continue conservative measure with taper and slowly add back in activity as tolerated. If there is no improvement or worsening of the condition, further diagnostics are necessary. X-ray films are usually the initial imaging study; they have only average benefit for exact diagnosis and location, but are used to rule out gross deformities. Depending on these results, MRI, myelogram, or discogram may be useful. Lab work such as CBC, ESR, alkaline phosphatase, and calcium are also indicated at this appointment if there is lack of progress.

Test usage and limitations

Toe-walking test is used to evaluate low back pain, if patient is unable to toe walk, this suggests a problem at the level of S1. Heel walking assesses function at L5. Limitations to both of these would be patient coordination or gait-disturbance from an unrelated source. Patellar and Achilles reflexes should be assessed for and neurological and musculoskeletal evaluation. Decreased patellar and normal Achilles reflex suggests a disturbance at L5. Reflex testing is limited in elderly patients and diabetics. The straight-leg test evaluates nerve entrapment at any lumbar level. Poor flexibility, tight hamstrings, and hip and pelvic disorders limit this test.

Lumbar spinal orthoses

Use of lumbar spinal orthoses is controversial. It is recommended to evaluate the use of these with evidence-based medicine and on a case-by-case basis, making careful patient selection. Elastic belts are often wide based with Velcro attachment at the front; they may have loose-fitting shoulder straps. These do not restrict range of motion and are not thought to prevent injury. However, elastic belts offer abdominal support and comfort in some. Lumbosacral corsets are a lace-up version of the above that may have hard plastic supports situated in them. They restrict range of motion minimally. Rigid orthoses are designed to prevent or limit flexion and extension but do not have an affect on rotation. All spinal orthoses should be used on a limited basis, in the acute phase only, as dependence on them weakens musculature.

Lumbar spine vs. cervical spine disorders

Low back pain is one of the top reasons that people seek medical care; furthermore, lumbar spine pain cause the most missed work days of any medical condition. The lumbar spine is surrounded by more structures such as ribs organs and pelvis and has much major postural and structural muscle groups to protect it. The cervical vertebrae are much smaller with only surrounding muscles and tendons to protect it. Given the smaller size of the cervical vertebrae, the spinal canal in this region is also much smaller. Therefore, injuries and degeneration in this area are often noticed sooner. Both the cervical and lumbar spine can have similar disorders including: herniated discs, spinal stenosis, spinal spondylosis and osteoarthritis.

Low back pain treatment options

When conservative measures fail, the patient may need long-term narcotic analgesic that may be better managed by a pain specialist. Pain specialists, often anesthesiologists, also may perform epidural steroid injections. Internal or external placement of spinal stimulation leads is also an option, to increase fusion likelihood in nonsurgical candidate or in a failed spinal fusion. If these fail, patient may be a surgical candidate. Surgical options include: vertebral spinal fusion, decompression of compresses nerves, laminectomy, disc excision, and a newer procedure called interdiscal electrothermal annuloplasty. These may be used in combination depending on the patient diagnosis.

Osteophyte formation in the cervical spine area

With large osteophyte formation anteriorly, impingement upon esophagus can cause difficulty and painful swallowing. If an osteophyte develops laterally, it can press upon the vertebral artery. Pressure on the vertebral artery can affect the vestibular system causing vertigo and ear ringing, it can also cause visual disturbance. With nerve impingement from osteophytes or cervical degeneration, radicular symptoms can be present in the upper extremities. Interruption at the C5-C6 level can cause pain in the biceps and pectoralis muscle. Pressure on nerve roots at the C6-C7 level causes tenderness over the triceps.

Spinal pain or spinal surgery considerations

The goal of teaching a patient with back pain proper body mechanics is to limit or avoid twisting, especially of the lumbar spine. So in the case of exiting a car effort must be made to keep body and spine in alignment at all times. From the forward facing position, the patient should slowly maneuver the body so that both feet can be placed on the ground (outside of the car) at the same time, while the body is also outward facing. With both feet on the ground, patient should place one hand on the opened car door and the other on the seat or doorframe. Hand placement is to help patients push themselves up. Try to keep forward bending to a minimum.

Nerve impingement at L5 and S1

The patient with pressure on the nerve roots at the level of L5 will have weakness with dorsiflexion of their foot and of their great toe. Difficulty with dorsiflexion or the push-off phase of walking is actually secondary to weakness in the calf musculature (gastronemius). They may also experience numbness or decreased sensation on the dorsal aspect of their foot. If S1 nerve roots are affected, the patient will complain of or demonstrate weakness with plantar flexion. They may have numbness on the lateral foot with S1 impingement. Furthermore, S1 nerve root pressure will yield a decreased Achilles reflex.

Nerve impingement at C6 and C7

These two cervical nerve roots are most commonly impinged upon:
C6 – This is a commonly affected area with neck injury or degeneration. The patient may complain of pain and decreased sensation that radiates down the arm and into

the thumb. Complaints or findings of muscle weakness in the biceps and the musculature responsible for extension of the wrist are common. The forearm or brachioradialis reflex will be decreased.

C7 – Pressure on this nerve causes complaints of pain and/or numbness that travels the length of the arm distally, to the third finger. A common finding on physical exam may be decreased triceps reflex.

Load-shifting knee braces

A load-shifting brace may be used in the patient with osteoarthritis. It is best utilized in an individual with unilateral (medial or lateral joint) compartment disease. It may be considered in the patient that has failed conservative treatment measures and is too young for total knee replacement or unicompartment arthroplasty. It is a brace with a rigid and lightweight frame that places either lateral or medial stress to the knee, to shift the load off of the affected side. Decreased pain and ease of use are some benefits that the patient reports. The braces are generally durable and patient compliance is good. One draw back is the cost.

Spinal discs

Spinal discs are the cushions in between our spinal vertebrae. Spinal discs are responsible for much of the shock absorption of our daily activities. The disc is composed of two main components: annulus fibrosus and nucleus pulposus. The annulus fibrosus is the outer portion comprised of collagen. The nucleus pulposus is the contained within the annulus fibosus and is gelatinous and primarily composed of water. Over time the gelatinous material becomes dehydrated and loses its volume through dehydration and compression. Neither component contains any blood or blood supply, therefore, it is not able to repair itself if it is damaged, compressed or dislocated (disc bulge).

Cervical traction

Mechanical cervical traction is widely used. It can be utilized in the home of the patient (with adequate instruction) or in the hospital setting. When used in the home environment, the goal is generally to reduce pain and provide comfort in an acute injury or acute flare of chronic injury. Results vary as to the success of cervical traction in reducing pain. In the hospital setting, mechanical cervical traction is primarily used for immobilization either pre or postsurgically. In the case of a trauma patient, cervical traction may be applied to immobilize the neck while stabilizing other injuries.

Cervical collars

Immobilization of the neck or cervical spine is the purpose of a cervical collar. It is also used to reduce pain and aid in recovery postsurgically. It is used for a number of nonsurgical conditions including: osteoarthritis, cervical spondylosis and whiplash injuries. Soft cervical collars and various rigid cervical spine collars are available. Soft neck collars are more often recommended for daytime use and allow for slightly more range of motion. Rigid collars are more likely to be used at night and postsurgically. If being used as an acute treatment, it is recommended that it only be used for a limited number of days. Long-term treatment with a soft collar can limit range of motion and weaken neck muscles.

Important terms

Distal interphalangeal joint: also known as the DIP joint, is the finger joint furthest or most distal from the body or wrist.
Proximal interphalangeal joint: also known as the PIP joint is the finger joint closest or more proximal to the wrist/body. This may also be known as the "middle joint" of

the finger. Note: the thumb has only one interphalangeal joint designated as the IP joint, distal or proximal designations are not needed on the thumb.

Metacarpophalangeal joint: also known as the MCP joint, is the finger joint that connects the metacarpal bones (hand bones) to the phalanges (finger bones). It is proximal to the PIP and DIP joints.

Heberden's nodes: bony growth at the DIP joint, seen in osteoarthritis. They are rarely painful and not progressive.

Bouchard's nodes: bony nodule growth at the PIP joint, seen in osteoarthritis.

Pronation: Used to refer to movements at the elbow (forearm) and wrist. Pronation is sometimes used to define movement of the ankle, although at this joint it can be synonymous with eversion. Pronation is the movement of the wrist and/or elbow that allows the palm of the hand to be facedown.

Supination: Used to refer to movements at the elbow (forearm) and wrist. Occasionally it will be used to describe ankle movements but is synonymous with ankle inversion. Supination is the movement of the wrist and/or elbow that ends-in and allows the palm of the hand to be face-up.

MTP joint: metatarsal phalangeal joint. This is the joint at the base of the toes, where the toe meets the foot. Main movements are flexion and extension. MTP joint identification is preceded by a number identifier to indicate which toe base is being discussed. For example, the first MTP joint is that of the great toe.

Hallux valgus: describes lateral deviation (toes pointing outward, while foot is in neutral/forward position) of the toes, specifically at the MTP joint and usually most prominent at the first MTP. It is often called "bunion".

Hallux rigidus: MTP (usually great toe) stiffness and osteoarthritis. This usually coexists with hallux valgus.

Spondylolisthesis: the forward dislocation of one vertebra on another, usually L5 on the sacrum. This can be from degeneration, disease, birth defect or trauma. On x-ray it looks like a "step off" in vertebral alignment.

Herniated nucleus pulposus: more commonly termed herniated disc or bulging disc. This can also be secondary to disease. The disc bulges through the spinal canal, narrowing it and putting pressure on spine and nerves exiting the column.

Spinal stenosis: narrowing of the spinal canal largely due to degeneration, although it can be congenital or pathological (as in a herniated disc).

Trauma

Cast instructions

The cast, in most cases, should be kept dry. Describe methods for keeping the cast dry while bathing, such as placing a plastic bag over the cast for showering or bathing. Remind the patient that the skin areas at the ends of the cast should be closely monitored; the rough edges may be filed with an emery board only. Instruct patient never to stick anything down into or under the cast to scratch and itch – if an object gets caught inside the cast, serious skin damage or infection can occur. To relieve an itch, the patient can point a hair dryer (on low and cool) into the end of it.

Remind the patient to always alert medical care personal in the event of tightness or increasing pain within the cast or numbness, color change, or temperature change in the areas at the distal end of the cast, and to follow up immediately if the cast is too loose or if it becomes cracked.

Describe methods of relieving pain and preventing swelling: elevating the cast above the heart and using ice packs over the cast. Also remind the patient not to forget to exercise the body on either side of the cast (move fingers and toes).

Paris vs. fiberglass casting

Both plaster of Paris and fiberglass are widely used, not only for casts but for splints as well. Factors in deciding which agent to use include: cost, physician comfort/familiarity, joint being immobilized, injury being treated and patient type. Plaster of Paris may be slightly cheaper; it molds well but is slightly heavier and has a much longer "setting" or drying time. This increased drying time and weight may not be ideal, for example, in a child in an outpatient setting, with an upper extremity injury. Fiberglass is slightly more expensive, comes in different colors, molds well, is lightweight and drying time can be as little as five minutes. It is also more water resistant. Due to the wider weave, the edges can be more abrasive and fiberglass tends to produce slightly more heat with application.

Bone types

Long bones: these are longer than they are wide. They consist of a shaft (diaphysis) and head (epiphyses). Examples of long bones are the humerus and femur. Short bones: these are cubical in shape. They are largely composed of spongy bone. Examples of short bones are the carpals in the wrist. Flat bones: thin and flat with slight curvature. They contain mostly compact bone. Examples include the skull bones. Irregular bones: these are bones that do not fit in the above classifications. They are composed mostly of spongy bone with thin compact outer layer. Examples of irregular bones include vertebrae and the bones that make up the pelvic girdle.

Long bone anatomy

A typical long bone, such as the humerus and femur, has two main components. The first component is the diaphysis that makes up the long shaft part of the bone. The outer portion is made of compact bone. The inner layer is made of marrow. The second main component of long bone is the epiphyses. The epiphyses are at either end of a typical long bone. The epiphyses are composed of an outer compact layer of bone and an inner core of spongy bone. A membrane lines both the diaphysis and epiphyses externally, called the periosteum. The periosteum contains a rich supply of nerve fibers, lymph and blood vessels.

Musculoskeletal injury and trauma

Injury from accidents is ranked fourth for cause of death. Traumatic injury from accidents leaps to the leading cause of death in the 35 and under age group. If the accident is not fatal, it ranks second in missed workdays. Accounting for a large percentage of traumatic musculoskeletal injury are motor vehicle accidents, occupational accidents, gunshots, falls and injuries sustained while operating power tools or machinery. Furthermore, a large number of traumatic injury results in bone fractures. Risk-taking behavior, especially seen in male teens and young adults, contributes to orthopedic injury. Other factors have been identified as contributors to traumatic injury, including: race, alcohol and substance abuse, socioeconomic standing, age, and geographic location. Education does not seem to be a factor.

Describing and classifying fractures

The first descriptive component of a fracture is location. This can include terms like: distal, proximal, lateral, and numbering like in phalanges and tarsals (3rd, 4th, and etc.). Location can also describe the portion of bone involved (epiphyses and diaphysis). The second classifier is a description of the fracture line itself, such as: spiral, oblique, comminuted, segmented, compressed, and transverse. Thirdly, describe the displacement of the fracture or its fragments. Examples of classifying displacement are: non-displaced, angulated, distracted or simply displaced. The fourth and final component of fracture classification is describing the condition of the soft-tissue surrounding the break as open or closed.

Predisposition to fractures

There are many different factors that could put patients at risk of fractures. Biological factors that contribute to the risk of bony fracture include age and type of bone involved. With increasing age, bone structure becomes less dense and more susceptible to injury. With type of bone, some bones are better equipped to handle different stresses and forces without injury. Extrinsic factors that predispose a person to bony fracture are: amount of force applied, angle of force applied, and duration of force. A behavioral factor that predisposes a patient to fracture is participating in adrenalin-seeking activities such as skydiving, rock-climbing and motor cross.

Fracture-healing factors

Skeletal maturity decreases healing; furthermore, an immature skeleton increases rate and success of healing. A single bone fracture has a better prognosis than multi-bone fractures. Transverse fractures have better outcome than oblique fractures. Significant displacement that affects surrounding soft tissue has an increased healing time. Thoracic spine fractures heal more effectively than unstable lumbar and cervical spine fractures. Fractures involving a joint surface are more unstable and difficult to treat. A fracture that has a nearby-unaffected bone for support has a good prognosis, as the unaffected bone adds stability and acts as a natural splint.

Knee injuries in motor vehicle accidents

The first possible injury is the 'dashboard fracture' that is a fracture of the rim of the acetabulum. The acetabulum is the socket and joint that contacts the femoral head. The fracture is caused by the impact of the femoral head. The second is a patellar fracture, from the force of the kneecap on the dash itself. Thirdly, the posterior cruciate ligament in the knee is often torn. The fracture types at the acetabulum and patella are usually comminuted. Possible, but less likely would be a stellate fracture of the acetabulum and patella.

Pelvic girdle fractures

The straddle fracture cause by, just as the name applies, forcefully falling on an object in the straddled position. This can be cause by coming down on a gymnastic bar, bike seat or being partially bucked from a horse. This injury usually transversely fractures the superior and inferior pubic rami and usually bilaterally. The dashboard fracture is caused by an automobile accident in which the knee hits the dashboard and that force progresses through the femur to the acetabulum (the bony structure that holds the femoral head) of the hip. The force of the femoral head against this socket or joint causes the fracture itself.

Gustilo-Anderson classification system

The Gustilo-Anderson classification system is used to describe and rate the level of soft tissue injury in open fractures. It classifies soft tissue injury into 6 levels. These levels are: Type I, II, III, IIIA, IIIB, and IIIC. Type I describes soft tissue damage that is minimal (<1 cm) and no signs of a crush mechanism. This level of soft tissue damage is usually seen in simple linear fractures. The levels progress through minor soft tissue involvement to level IIIC, which has a high rate of amputation, as blood supply is grossly damaged.

Nonunion

Exact definitions for nonunion remain unclear. Nonunion describes a fracture that does not heal or has delayed healing. The time frames for this definition are what remain controversial. It is thought that a fracture can be described as a nonunion if there is no evidence of bony callus (healing) formation on x-rays after 5 months of appropriate immobilization and treatment. Risk factor for lack of healing after 5 months are: smoking, infection, malnutrition, no steroidal anti-inflammatory medication, improper immobilization techniques, noncompliance with immobilization, and poor blood supply within the injured bone.

'Mallet Finger' injuries

Trauma to the end of an extended finger, causing a forceful flexion, avulses the extensor tendon from its attachment site. A portion of this attachment site, the dorsal base of the distal phalanx, may itself be avulsed with the extensor tendon. The third finger is most frequently involved, since it is the longest. This is often described as a "jammed finger". Treatment includes a dorsal splint (holding the DIP joint in full extension) for about 8 weeks. After the 8 weeks, it is recommended to continue with a nighttime only splint.

Internal fracture fixation devices

Screws: this is one of the most common fixation devices and comes in many forms. Depending on the type, they can be tapped or threaded into the bone. They can be placed directly into bone, but are more commonly used with a plate.

Plate: this is held in place by screws and is usually used along the diaphysis of the bone.

Wires and pins: these are usually made of stainless steel and are good for small bone. They can be pulled through the skin for removal.

Cortical screws: contain tight threading.

Cancellous screws: only partially threaded with wide thread.

Malleolar screws: partially threaded with narrow threading.

Nail & sliding screw-plate: used for hip replacements.

Contraindications for open reduction

The first contraindication for open fracture reduction is infection. Infection in the bone (osteomyelitis) is the most obvious, but infection elsewhere in the body should prevent open reduction. Secondly, loss of bone density such as that seen in osteopenia and osteoporosis is not conducive to open reduction. Thirdly, if bony fragments at the fracture site are too small for fixation devices, open reduction is not indicated. Fourthly, open reduction should not be performed with limited surrounding soft tissue, such as in severe burns. Finally, open reduction in contraindicated in the patient with multiple uncontrolled comorbidities.

Limb amputation indications

Amputation is indicated if the injury sustained to the bone was a crush injury in which the limb did not have a blood supply for greater than six hours, secondary to the trauma. If the main nerve supplying the limb is completely severed in the trauma, then amputation is necessary. The decision for amputation is also based on the other trauma sustained. If there are multiple injuries, amputation is probable. If other injuries include areas distal to the site, amputation is recommended. Other factors to take into account are recovery time in relation to procedure itself and in relation to other injuries. Furthermore, consider age, health, occupation and prognosis of alternative treatments.

5 stages of fracture healing

Stage one is the inflammatory response with hematoma development, lasting up to 3 days. Stage two sees tissue granules break-up the hematoma and cartilaginous tissue forms, through the second week. Stage three continues to see the tissue mature and callus development through 6 weeks. In stage four the callus reaches to provide continuity to the fracture site, this will eventually be replaced by bone, through 24 weeks. The fifth and final stage continues through the first year, the bone strengthens to meet the requirements for movement and force application.

Traumatically injured limbs

Initial assessment of a traumatically injured limb includes visualization. It is important to note and describe the soft tissue injury, location, and color of intact surrounding skin and how this compares to color of skin distal to the injury. Using the opposite and unaffected limb for comparison is helpful, if this is an option. Next, note the temperature, pulses, edema, and neurologic function (sensation and reflexes) of the limb proximal and distal to the site of trauma and compared to opposite extremity. Be aware of signs of prior chronic disease by looking for non-accident related ulceration, check for hair distribution, health of finger/toenails.

MESS

MESS stands for Mangles Extremity Severity Score. It is a system used to help medical providers determine if amputation or attempts at limb salvage should be undertaken. The scoring system is based on four areas. The first area to be scored is the amount of injury sustained to bone and soft tissue. The second area determines how much the blood supply to the area had been affected and for how long. The third component is the amount of shock sustained by the patient. Fourth and final is age of the patient. Consideration and scoring of these four factors is paramount. A score of >7 means amputation is probable, and attempts at salvaging the limb are not likely to be successful.

Types of amputation

Closed amputation: this is the most common form of amputation. However, this is not often used in trauma cases. This procedure involves use and preparation of skin flaps to close over the amputation site. Often, this allows preparation for prosthesis fitting later.
Open amputation: this is the most common form of amputation after traumatic injury to a limb or when there is severe infection. In this procedure, the wound and fracture site is left open for secondary closure later. To prevent skin from retracting, traction may be used so there is a skin flap available to cover the area at time of closure. If skin cover is not available, grafting is necessary.
Autoamputation: a procedure used for the digits only. Also used in patients that are not surgical candidates. The digit is frozen or gangrenous area is allowed to separate itself after a necrotic boundary is established.

Evaluating a traumatic limb

Transcutaneous oxygen pressure determination: this test is considered noninvasive and is commonly used. Some consider this the best test for predicting healing outcome of an amputation.
Doppler ultrasound: this test is a noninvasive test that visualizes tissue and blood flow to an extremity. This is a cost effective test.
Laser Doppler flowmetry: this is a noninvasive test to evaluate blood flow through the arteries and veins of extremities.
Ankle-brachial index (ABI): a noninvasive test that measure blood pressures of the upper and lower extremities at rest and/or after exercise. An ABI of <1 indicates narrowing of a vessel in the leg.
Angiorgram: this is a commonly used invasive method. This is a widely used test but is not prognostic for amputation healing. It is a better predictor of artery reconstruction or repair.

Amputee patient concerns

Nursing and a multi-medical team approach is important for successful for all phases of amputation. Patient education is important through all phases. Presurgically it is important to discuss the benefits and necessities of amputation versus limb salvage. Establishing physical therapy in all phases is important for successful rehab. Connecting patients with counselors and support groups is important for coping and self-image issues. Pain management and pain management options should be discussed and implemented. Stump care should be reviewed, as well as signs and symptoms of complications. Prosthetic options and stump preparation of prosthetic devices should be discussed. All interventions should have the common goal of returning the amputee to independent functioning with minimal pain.

Phantom limb pain (PLP) is pain experienced by an amputee; often developing up to three months post surgery. It is a sensation of pain felt in the limb that has been amputated. It is common in all amputees over age 6, and sometimes more severe in above-the-knee amputees or traumatic amputees that were in a great deal of presurgical pain. In a large percentage of amputees, PLP is self-limiting and can be helped with medication, desensitization, electrical stimulation, counseling, hypnosis, acupuncture and nerve block if needed. Phantom limb sensation (PLS) is similar to PLP, except the sensations of the missing limb are not painful. Sensations such as itching, tingling and temperature variants can be felt PLS. The telescoping phenomenon is the sensation of the amputated limb slowly being retracted into the stump. In telescoping, the sensations of the great toe, thumb and index finger are the last to "disappear" into the stump.

Stump care is important for reduction of pain, infection, complications and prosthetic fitting. Once daily washing is important. Excessive washing is discouraged as this facilitates dryness and skin breakdown. Stress thorough drying and inspection prior to application of shrink-wraps or prosthetics. If patient cannot visualize the end of the stump, educating the family members of caregivers is equally important. Evaluation includes any changes in skin including sores, redness or warmth to touch or changes in sensation. Daily message of the stump is important for reducing adhesions and promoting desensitization. Infection management must be discussed. If there is a break in the stump skin, instruct to air this area for at least one hour, four times daily. Shrinkage wraps should be washed and/or replaced daily.

The purpose of all stump-shrinking devices is to reduce swelling post-amputation and prepare the limb for prosthetic fitting. Ace bandages are the first type, widely used, cost-effective, widely available, and can easily be removed for limb inspection. Disadvantages of Ace bandages are they are not great for shaping the limb and application is dependent on patient's ability and compliance. The second method of stump shrinkage is shrinker socks. These are pre-made, can be easily removed and allow adequate pressure and shaping. They are easy to apply and thus helpful for compliance. Disadvantages include: moderate cost, size limitations (especially for the very large or very small), and the need for frequent size changes as limb shrinks. Finally, rigid dressing is used. This is essentially a cast placed on the limb. This allows for control of edema, prosthetic shaping, protection, early weight bearing and good compliance.

Wrist fractures

Colles' fracture is a break of the distal radius. The mechanism is usually falling on an outstretched hand, or bracing oneself against the dashboard in an auto accident. This fracture can be accompanied by distal ulnar fracture, scaphoid fracture, it can be angulated, displaced and with multiple bony fragments. Fracture is confirmed with x-ray. In most cases, immobilization, with or without closed reduction, is recommended with a sugar-tong splint. Ice, elevation and anti-inflammatory medication is recommended for the first 72 hours. Encourage movement of shoulder and fingers. Repeat x-ray in one week, if fracture is stable and swelling has stopped, apply short-arm cast. Cast should be worn for 4-6 weeks with intermittent evaluation and cast-care instructions. Because of close proximity to the median nerve, complications from improper immobilization or poor healing may result in carpal tunnel syndrome.

Humerus fractures

Diaphyseal or shaft fracture: most common near the middle of the shaft. Closed reduction is common with cast or splint and sling in minor cases. If open reduction is indicated, plate and screws are usually placed.
Anatomic neck fracture: break is at the metaphysis of the humerus. Sling application and rehabilitation program is the common treatment.
Surgical neck fracture: this fracture is below the anatomic neck or below the metaphysis. Severe angulation is usually seen due to its anatomical position. Treatment, therefore, includes closed reduction and sling application to maintain alignment.

Scaphoid fractures

The scaphoid bone is the most commonly broken carpal (wrist) bone. It is at the base of the thumb and the mechanism of injury is falling on an outstretched hand. Physical exam will include tenderness in the "anatomical snuff box". Initial x-ray may not show a fracture, but if history and physical exam suggests the possibility of a scaphoid fracture, it needs to be treated as such. Initial treatment includes immobilization with either a radial gutter splint or ventral splint with thumb extension. Repeat x-ray in 10-14 days and at that time consider short-arm cast with thumb spica. If the scaphoid is broken in the middle or proximal portion, open reduction and screw placement is possible.

Instruct patients on the slow healing time of this fracture and the importance of compliance with immobilization due to the high risk of nonunion and avascular necrosis of the bone.

Boxer's fractures

A Boxer's fracture is most commonly a fracture of the distal metacarpal head of the 5th digit; however, it may also be seen in the 4th digit. Evaluate the skin for laceration or deep abrasion, as the presence of these turns the fracture into an open fracture. Provide wound care and infection management accordingly. Physical exam will likely include swelling, bruising, and pain over the affected metacarpal. Patient may or may not be able to make a fist, when attempting this; you may notice malalignment (pointing more towards the thumb than the opposite hand) of the affected metacarpal. X-ray is diagnostic. If minimal angulation and displacement is present, place patient in an ulnar gutter splint extending distal to PIP joint of affected digit to just below the elbow. If deformity and displacement is significant, consider closed reduction. Splint should remain for 3 weeks with appropriate follow up and pain management.

Fracture emergency assessment

Initially the fractures take back seat to the stabilization of the multi-trauma patient. First evaluate and stabilize the airway and breathing, this may include cervical spine collar/board. Evaluate cardiovascular and shock status, options may include performing cardiopulmonary resuscitation, obtaining venous access, and/or providing fluids if appropriate. Obvious life-threatening injuries need to be addressed and stabilized first, any bleeding controlled, and immobilization via splinting of any suspected fractures. Evaluate neurovascular status of potential fracture sites. Splinting serves to stabilize the injury, prevent further damage, and reduce pain and bleeding while vital organ systems are being tended to. Once the patient's vitals have been stabilized, it is possible to start focused orthopedic assessment, definitive diagnostics, and treatment.

Anatomical snuff box

The anatomical snuffbox is visualized best on a patient when they have their thumb fully abducted and slightly extended (hitch-hikers position). It is the indented triangular compartment seen on the dorsal lateral hand at the base of the thumb. It is comprised of the abductor pollicis longus and extensor pollicis brevis that make up the anterior portion of the triangular area. The extensor pollicis longus makes up the posterior portion of the triangle. The distal radius makes up the base of the snuffbox triangle. The scaphoid carpal bone primarily makes the floor of the triangular anatomical snuffbox. The significance of this landmark is that the radial artery runs through here and a branch of the radial nerve. If any of the structures that make up this landmark are injured, especially the scaphoid bone, complications can ensue because of likely concurrent disruption of the radial artery.

Important Terms

Fracture: this describes a break in the bone itself. A fracture may or may not involve a joint surface. A fracture may be a full thickness or partial thickness fracture.

Dislocation: this is used to describe a complete disruption in a joint. The joint surface of both bones, no longer make contact with each other. Subluxation: this refers to an incomplete dislocation of a joint from its normal position. With a subluxation, there is still partial contact of the joint surfaces. This is sometimes referred to as a 'partial dislocation'.

Crush: this fracture mechanism is caused by a large stress on a small area. These usually result in multiple break lines and severe soft tissue damage. A few examples of this would be a sledgehammer missing the mark and coming down on a finger/wrist or a heavy suspended mass falling on a foot/leg.

Compression: this fracture mechanism is sustained when there is a large axial loading force. Compression fractures are most often noted in the vertebrae. An example would be a fall from a moderate height, and the person landing on their feet or buttocks.

Stress: this fracture mechanism is one of the few that is not sustained by trauma or a one-time stress. A stress fracture can occur in normal bone with normal but repetitive activity that places a stress on this bone over time.

Angulation: this force mechanism causes the bony fragment to become broken transversely and then misaligned, usually in a v-shape. An example of this can be the same as that of a tapping force, when one uses their forearm to block a blow. However, the force to cause misalignment is usually greater than that of a tapping injury.

Rotational: the mechanism of this fracture causes a spiraling fracture line. This fracture often occurs in the arms or lower leg, and when seen in a child should raise the question of abuse.

Tapping: the mechanism of this fracture is sustained from a small force to a concentrated area. The bone absorbs this force and there may or may not be mild soft tissue display of the injury. An example of this would be a fracture of the forearm when blocking a hit with a fist or bat. This is also common on the lower leg after being kicked.

Penetrating: this fracture mechanism is caused by a large amount of force on a small area. The difference between this and a crush injury is the object of force is usually small also and soft tissue involvement is minimal. An example of this is a stab wound or gunshot wound.

Linear fracture: implies that the fracture forms a straight line through the bone. It does not, however, differentiate if this line is angled or horizontal.

Oblique fracture: describes a fracture line that travels at an angle through a bone.

Transverse fracture: describes a break that travels in a horizontal line through a bone. Therefore, a linear fracture can be transverse or oblique. This follows that a fracture should never simply be termed 'linear' without the more descriptive terms transverse or oblique accompanying it.

Avulsion fracture: this describes a break that displaces a portion of bone from it usual position. This is most likely to occur at the ends of bones, and thus the bone chip often affects the joint space.

Comminuted fracture: this is used to describe a fracture that results in greater than two bony fragments. This is often used to describe a crush injury.

Greenstick fracture: this fracture is usually the result of a lesser force and does not cause a full-thickness break. Only one side of the bone is affected, and therefore this is not a fracture associated with displacement.

Impacted fracture: this is a fracture in which a smaller portion of bone is forced or compressed into the larger portion of bone. This is sometimes called a telescope fracture.

Torus fracture: this fracture is commonly described as a buckle fracture. A buckle fracture is one in which the bone appears bowed and may not really appear broken at all. It is used to describe a bone that buckles on the side of impact, but does not disrupt the other side of the bone. It may also be termed 'incomplete fracture'.

Occult fracture: this is a fracture that cannot immediately be recognized on x-ray. It is either hidden or difficult to discern from normal structures and lines. This can often be seen via x-ray 2-4 weeks after the original films or injury, by the new bone formation.

Autogenous bone: this is a bone graft taken from the patient, usually from the iliac crest. It is useful for small bony defects, but has a high rate of complications.

Allographic bone: this is where cadaver bone is injected into a fracture site. It may be beneficial in larger bone defects, but has an increased risk of infection.

Synthetic bone substitutes: substitutes include ceramics and sea coral. These are most successful when injected into large fractures that have already been surgically stabilized.

Bioactive cells and proteins: many of these substances are still being studied and utilized in medical trials. They show benefit for nonunion fractures, but are very expensive.

Sports Injuries

Many sports-related injuries are preventable. Preventable injuries include: poor conditioning, poor technique, faulty or improper equipment, improper footwear, inadequate warm-up and stretching, and too early of a return from a previous injury. Even if all of these preventable criteria are met, there is still room for accidental or non-preventable sport injuries. Many sports injuries are minor sprains and strains and a large percentage are non-surgical. Rarely do sport injuries include brain or spinal cord injuries, but these should always be considered in evaluation of an athletic injury, especially with traumatic collisions seen in contact sports.

It is important, when treating sports injuries, to always remember you are treating the whole patient not just an athlete. Diagnostic and treatment considerations are to be made on what is best for the person's life, not just their sport and team. Special populations include: the very young athlete, the older athlete, and women. When dealing with little-leaguers, you are dealing with an immature skeleton. With older recreational sport participants, considerations such as decreased bone density, cardiovascular changes, and decline in muscle mass must be taken into account. In the competitive female athlete, endurance training may result in amenorrhea, which may result in decreased bone density and increased likelihood of stress fractures.

Shin splints

Shin splints are an injury that results from stress on the tibia. The medical term for this condition is: medial tibial stress syndrome. This condition is most frequently seen in runners; however, it can appear in any sport. Conditions that may make one susceptible to shin splints are repetitive heavy impact on hard surfaces (basketball, tennis) and training too hard or too long with poor stretching. The risk of developing shin splint is increase with poor or improper-fitting shoes. Those with 'flat feet' are more likely to develop shin splints.

Treatment of shin splints is primarily rest. However, these can take along time heal, and athletes often become impatient with this treatment. After the initial rest period, an ongoing stretching program and ruling out a stress fracture, the athlete may slowly add in activity. Initially, activity should be low impact and short duration, building up to their previous activity level as pain and injury allows. Ice, compression wrappings and orthotics may be used, not only for treatment, but for prevention and self-care as well. Prevention also includes proper cool-down, stretching and elevation of legs after workout. Changing footwear out at least every 6 months or 400 miles, helps prevent many injuries. Consider cross training to include lower impact workout like swimming and bicycling. Strength training, building muscles up to take stress off of the bones, joints and ligaments can also be helpful.

Sprains and strains

The biggest point of differentiation in sprains and strains is the presence or absence of trauma. A traumatic force to a joint causes a sprain. This force temporarily moves the joint out of its usual limits or motion. A sprain causes varying degrees of damage to ligaments. Ligament can be stretched, partially torn, or completely torn. The degree of ligament damage defines the severity of the sprain. Most common joints to be sprained are the ankle, knee and wrist. A strain is an injury sustained without contact or trauma. Strains usually happen when a muscle group is overstretched or overcontracted. A strain involves tendon or muscle. Again, tendons and muscles can be stretched or torn. Strains can involve any muscle/tendon group in the body.

"Weekend warrior"

Weekend warrior is a term commonly used to describe the person that does not exercise routinely during the week, but is involved in various levels of physical activity during the weekend. They often place one-week worth of activities into 1-2 days. This person is often middle-aged and an x-athlete. Weekend participation may be recreational or competitive. The weekend warrior often does not stretch, warm-up or cool-down properly. The above factors predispose the weekend warrior to sport injuries such as strains and tendonitis. Achilles tendonitis and tear is a common injury in weekend warriors participating in competitive contact or noncontact sports.

R.I.C.E

The acronym R.I.C.E stands for Rest, Ice, Compression, and Elevation. This is a common treatment recommendation for sport injuries. It is also a good patient education tool for self-care of minor sport injuries and strains. If this is not reducing the patient's symptoms after 48 hours, the patient should consider medical evaluation. The "Rest" component indicates reducing normal activity until pain lessens. Activity as tolerated or weight bearing as tolerated is often used when prescribing "Rest". Ice is recommended for initial and acute injury, especially within the first 72 hours of injury. Ice affected areas for no more than 20-minute intervals. Compression includes Ace bandages or air casts. This adds support and reduces swelling. Elevation also helps inflammation. Keep the injured body part elevated above the level of the heart whenever possible. Some add a "D" to this acronym, D-R.I.C.E. The "D" stands for drugs, specifically nonsteroidal anti-inflammatories and analgesics.

Achilles tendonitis

Achilles tendonitis occurs more frequently in individuals that have taken a break from physical activity and then suddenly participate at full speed. It can also occur in the conditioned athlete, but this is less frequent. Factors that predispose a person to develop Achilles tendonitis include: poor fitting footwear, overuse, inadequate stretching, tight or weak calf muscles, running on hard surfaces or hills, flat feet, sharp plant and pivot activities, or a combination of any of these factors. Prevention or risk-reduction includes altering or avoiding the above conditions. Strengthening with toe-raises is helpful. Cross training prevents excessive strain on one muscle group.

Treatment options for children vs. adults

Sport injuries in children cannot be treated the same as adult injuries. A child's immature bony structure predisposes them to many different injuries and outcomes. Sport injuries in children can range from minor to lifelong complication. An injury that would cause a sprain in an adult could very well break a child's bone. Children of the same age can vary greatly in their maturity and skill level when participating in competitive sports. This degree of variation in build, size, maturity and skill level puts children on the same playing field at increased risk for injury. The top five recreational and sporting activities that cause injury in children aged 5-14 are: bicycle injuries, basketball, football, playground equipment and batting sports (baseball and softball). Sport injuries in the adult age 25 and over are most common with the following activities: recreational sports (hiking, golf, bowling, and racquet sports), exercise, basketball, bicycling, and batting sports.

Sport injuries rehabilitation options

RICE is often prescribed and taught by the family practitioner, orthopedist and/or nurse. Along with range of motion and strengthening at physical therapy, the therapist may institute a number of modalities to enhance progress. Massage is one of these modalities. Either professional or self-massage helps stimulate blood flow to the injury site. Ultrasound also helps stimulate blood flow by high-frequency sound waves that produce deep heat to the affected area. Thermotherapy increases blood flow to the injury, but should not be used within the first 72 hours of injury. Thermotherapy includes: heating pads, microwavable rice bags, warm-water therapy, and heat lamps. Electrostimulation interferes with pain signals to the brain, from the site of injury. This relieves pain, reduces swelling and helps maintain muscle strength.

Tennis elbow

Tennis elbow is an overuse injury that affects the lateral epicondyle of the elbow, thus its medical name: lateral epicondylitis. It not only affects tennis players, but any athlete that repetitively or forcefully contracts the forearm muscles with elbow and wrist movements. This injury can affect those in throwing sports, most ball sports, and racquet sports. It may also be an occupational injury. Treatment includes: rest, ice, stretching, massage, strengthening, anti-inflammatory medications or injections, and use of splints/braces at the wrist and proximal forearm. Surgical treatment is rare. Prevention and self-care is the same as treatment measures but also includes learning proper technique and reducing racquet string tension.

Protective equipment

Protective equipment can refer to an item worn by the athlete or an external item in the sporting arena that reduces injury to the athlete. Contact sports such as football and hockey institute a number of personal protective gear: helmets, pads (rib, shoulder, knee, and wrist), and mouth guards. Soccer players use shin-guards. Boxers use gloves, kidney guards and sometimes headgear. Water sports may include life jackets and wet suits. Examples of external protective equipment are: wall pads, goal-post padding, goal-post attachment (soccer), spotters (weight training), and level playing surfaces (football, soccer, lacrosse, and etc. playing fields).

Ankle sprains

Ankle sprain is the most common sport injury. Ankle sprains are classified as first degree, second degree, or third degree sprains. First degree sprains are associated with mild pain and swelling, normal range of motion and ankle tests and minimal gait impairment. After treatment, return to activity should be no sooner than 10 days. Second degree ankle sprains are associated with moderate pain and swelling, decreased range of motion and positive findings in the ankle exam. After treatment and rehabilitation, return to sport should be after 2 weeks with ankle support wrap. Third degree ankle sprains have severe pain and swelling and all ankle tests are positive. Patient is usually unable to weight bear initially. Return to competition after treatment and rehabilitation should be no sooner than 4 weeks, with continued ankle bracing.

Golfer's elbow

Golfer's elbow is similar to tennis elbow except that it affects the medial aspect of the elbow. Its medical name is medial epicondylitis. Golfer's elbow can be seen in athletes that participate in golf, racquet sports, throwing sports and different occupations and hobbies. Any activity that includes forceful gripping coupled with repetitive wrist movement can cause this injury. Treatment of golfers elbow includes: rest, ice initially, heat after 72 hours, forearm brace or compression wrap, oral anti-inflammatory and analgesic medications, steroid injections, stretching and strengthening program, and gradual return to activity with technique review. Surgery is rarely required.

Turf toe

Turf toe is an injury to the joint capsule at the base of the great toe. It is caused by forceful hyperextension at this joint. The name implies artificial turf playing fields, as these do not have as much "give" and grip is sustained while body movement continues forward. Although this is a common football injury, it can occur in any sport that requires quick pivot and direction changes such as soccer and rugby. Treatment includes rest, avoid competitive sports for up to 6 weeks, ice, elevation, preventing excessive toe movement (change in footwear or toe splint insert), anti-inflammatories, and in severe cases wearing a walking boot.

Ankle sprain tests

Anterior drawer test: this test is used to assess the function of the anterior talofibular ligament. Stabilizing the lower leg and pulling the heel anteriorly perform this test. The drawer test is positive if there is significant laxity or a sharp endpoint is felt.
Talar tilt test: this test is used to assess the stability of the calcaneofibular ligament. This test is performed by stabilizing the lower leg with one hand and with the other hand on the heel, invert and evert ankle. The test is positive if there is significant

laxity compared to the unaffected ankle and if there is a tight endpoint in either direction.
Squeeze test: this test assess damage to the medial ankle compartment made up of several ligamentous structures. This test is positive if there is pain in the ankle when the middle of the tibia and fibula bones are squeezed together.

Plantar fasciitis

Plantar fasciitis is an injury to the fascia that makes up the arch and bottom of the foot. It attaches at the heel and toes. The attachment sites can become inflamed and painful for a variety of reasons. Athletes that experience this are commonly runners, ballerinas and aerobics participation. Nonathletic causes of plantar fasciitis are: extremes of foot arch, obesity, diabetics, age, pregnancy, occupations (standing long hours on hard floors), footwear with poor arch support, and arthritis. Treatment is nonsurgical and includes RICE, stretching, weight loss, orthotics and sometimes steroid injections.

Metatarsalgia

Metatarsalgia is a pain in the ball of the foot or the distal metatarsals. This is caused from repetitive or high-impact trauma to this area such as jumping, running on hard surfaces, poor footwear, and any activity that includes a forceful "push-off" phase. Due to the anatomy of the foot, the first and second metatarsals are most likely involved. With certain movements, the force on these bones can be almost 300% of a person's body weight. There are many factors that predispose a person to this sport injury. Changeable factors include: intense training seen in endurance athletes, poorly fitting shoes, and excessive body weight. Furthermore, endurance athletes are more prone to stress fractures, which can be seen in the metatarsals. Unchangeable predisposing factors for developing metatarsalgia are: age, high foot arch, hammertoe, bunions, and Morton' neuroma.

Shoulder injuries

"Thrower's shoulder," "pitcher's shoulder," and "swimmer's shoulder" are all terms used to describe rotator cuff (RTC) tendonitis often seen in baseball pitchers and competitive swimmers. The forceful and repetitive shoulder abduction and extreme external rotation cause this injury. These movements cause the tendons of the RTC to be pinched between the head of the humerus and the rim of the posterior glenoid (shoulder joint). Treatment, self-care, and prevention include RICE, slings, stretching, strengthening, technique evaluation, anti-inflammatory and analgesic medication, steroid injections, and if conservative treatment fails surgery may be considered. Surgical options include arthroscopy and open surgical repair.

Heat concerns for the athlete

Heat cramps, heat exhaustion and heatstroke in an athlete are all concerns for the athlete. Heat cramps are cause by sweating which causes depletion of sodium chloride. This is most often experienced in the abdomen and legs. Treatment involves electrolyte replacement with sport drinks. Heat exhaustion occurs when the athlete's bodily response to heat and sweating is abnormal. In this athlete, sweating triggers the peripheral vessels to constrict and the core body temperature to rise. The athlete with heat exhaustion will be cool and clammy and pale on the outside. Treatment includes drinking cool sports drinks, rest, and application of external cooling devices. Heatstroke in an athlete is a severe and life-threatening condition. This occurs when the body's cooling mechanisms fail such as sweating and dysfunctional circulation. The athlete's skin will be dry, red and hot, vitals abnormal, and various levels of consciousness may be observed. Get the patient to emergency medical intervention immediately, while externally cooling the body and starting IV fluids.

Anterior cruciate ligament injury

Treatment options for anterior cruciate ligament (ACL) injury include nonsurgical and surgical options. Nonsurgical treatments may be initiated and if progress is poor, surgical options may be considered. Nonsurgical options are undertaken under the following circumstances: knee is stable with daily activities, a secondary injury to the knee is absent, and if the person will no longer be participating in high-impact sports. Treatment would then include RICE initially, aggressive physical therapy program, ongoing home exercise program, activity modification, and use of knee brace with certain activities. If the above criteria for nonsurgical treatment are not met, the athlete proceeds to surgical intervention. The goal of surgery is to restore knee stability and prevention of future knee injury upon resuming sport participation. A lengthy rehabilitation program follows surgical reconstruction of the ACL.

Injury of the anterior cruciate ligament (ACL) in the knee of an athlete is most often sustained when the foot is planted and body momentum causes the knee to twist forcefully. Another common mechanism of this injury is when the foot it planted, knee externally rotated and a lateral force is applied to the knee. Clinical diagnostic tests for ACL injury are Lachman's test and the pivot shift test. The Lachman's test is done by applying posterior pressure on the distal thigh and pulling the proximal lower leg anteriorly while the knee is slightly flexed. This test is positive if there is increase laxity compared to the uninjured knee. The pivot shift test is started in extension; with foot internally rotated and lateral pressure at the knee the knee is flexed. This test is positive if subluxation occurs.

Meniscal injury

Meniscal injuries usually happen with a twisting and compression type of force. Often times they are not an isolated injury, due to the mechanism.

Meniscal tears often coexist with ACL injuries. The patient with meniscal damage classically complains of painful popping and locking. Diagnosis is made with a positive McMurray test and MRI. The McMurray test is started with the knee in the maximal comfortable flexion position. The foot is then held in external rotation and the knee slowly straightened. If this maneuver elicits a pop or pain, it is positive.

Posterior cruciate ligament injury

A posterior cruciate ligament (PCL) knee injury can be sustained when the knee is forcefully hyperextended. PCL damage can also occur when a flexed knee sustains an anterior force such as falling onto the bent knee. Clinical exams that would be consistent with a PCL injury or tear include the posterior drawer test and the quadriceps active drawer test. Both test for laxity and are best used when compared to the unaffected knee. An MRI may be necessary for diagnosis, this can also show other structure damage, as often occurs with PCL injury.

Osteochondritis dissecans

Osteochondritis dissecans (OD) most commonly affects the knee, but is also seen in the elbow (pitchers) and ankle. It is a condition in which there is a lack of bony blood supply near the joint surface, eventually causing bone deterioration. Its incidence is more common in teenage males; however, OD is increasing in the female population due to increased participation of females in competitive sports. The exact cause of OD is unclear; however it is theorized that OD is secondary to repetitive small traumas that eventually cause fracture or wearing away of joint cartilage.

Conservative treatment of osteochondritis dissecans is usually the most successful. This includes resting and immobilizing the joint. At least six weeks of rest and reduced activity are recommended before return to full sport participation. Use of nonsteroidal anti-inflammatory and/or analgesic medication is often needed. Physical therapy with stretching, strengthening and low-impact cardiovascular emphasis is recommended. Surgery is only a consideration if lack of improvement with conservative measures persists beyond six months. The main complication of osteochondritis dissecans, if left untreated or inadequately treated, is the early development of degenerative osteoarthritis in the affected joint.

"Little Leaguers Elbow"

Younger athletes that forcefully and repetitively throw are prone to this injury, just as the name implies. This is essentially a tendonitis of the elbow, as the forceful pull of the tendons of the elbow joint are repetitively stressed. In severe cases, these tendons can be pulled from the bone with or without bony avulsion. The young athlete usually complains of medial elbow pain and/or knot, locking and decreased range of motion. Treatment is usually conservative with RICE and physical therapy to strengthen surrounding musculature. Surgery is only an option in the older athlete.

"Burners" or "Stingers"

A stinger or burner is most often described in context with contact sports such as football. This injury happens with one of three mechanisms. The first is when the nerves between the shoulder and neck are forcefully stretched when the shoulder is forced in an inferior direction and the neck is simultaneously forcefully laterally flexed to the contralateral side. The second mechanism of a stinger injury is when the head is forced to the side, pinching the nerve on that same side. Finally, an athlete can get a stinger when the nerves are bruised from a direct hit above the clavicle.

Osgood-Schlatter disease

Osgood-Schlatter disease (OSD) is a disorder thought to be caused by repetitive minor injury to the attachment site of the patellar tendon on the tibial tuberosity. It is more common in males and often first noticed around the time of a growth spurt. It is also common in jumping sports and sports that require a great deal of plant-and-pivot and directional changes. The patient will complain of pain and swelling right at the tibial tubercle. There is often a palpable tibial tuberosity on exam, and this reproduces pain. Treatment is conservative and the disease is self-limiting and usually resolves upon skeletal maturity.

Shoulder dislocations

The shoulder is the most commonly dislocated joint in the body. The shoulder can dislocate as a result of a sports injury in which a force is applied to the shoulder, forcefully dislodging the humeral head from the shoulder socket. This can happen in three directions (anterior, posterior, and inferior). A shoulder dislocation can also result in injury to the surrounding support structures such as the ligaments. This is often why repeat injury and dislocation is common. Treatment for dislocated shoulder is relocation via closed reduction, often followed by immobilization. Physical therapy follows stabilization to strengthen surrounding musculature and prevent future dislocation.

Neuromuscular/Pediatric/Congenital

Duchenne's muscular dystrophy

Duchenne's muscular dystrophy is the most common type. This is genetic and most commonly seen in males between 2 and 6 years of age. Early symptoms include clumsiness, fatigue with walking, toe walking, and large calf muscles. Pelvic girdle is usually the first involved muscle group to display weakening. Exam may reveal positive Gower's sign and ankle reflexes greater than knee reflexes. Diagnostic tests include muscle biopsy, EMG testing, elevated CPK levels and MRI. Treatment involves physical therapy, education, leg braces and/or wheelchair, support groups for patient and family, weight control, and regular medical follow-up. Prognosis is poor beyond age 20.

Muscular dystrophy

Muscular dystrophy (MD) is a disorder of progressively weakening muscles. In later and severe stages of the disease, muscle fibers can be replaced by fat. This replacement of muscle fibers by fat, not only affects the musculoskeletal system, but vital organs such as the heart as well. There are several different types of this disorder ranging in severity and body portion that it affects. Treatment is palliative and it is important to institute an aggressive program of self-care and patient and family education. Early signs and symptoms of MD are significant incoordination, clumsiness, balance difficulties, muscle weakness, difficulty with stairs, and problems getting to the standing position.

Cerebral palsy

Cerebral palsy is a neuromuscular disorder that affects a person's ability to control their muscles. This disorder is not progressive. A child is often born with this disorder, but it may not manifest until three years of age. There are several causes of cerebral palsy including: abnormal development in utero, infection in mother during pregnancy, traumatic birth, premature delivery, severe newborn jaundice and severe infant infections. Head injuries later in childhood can also cause cerebral palsy. There are still many theories as to the exact cause of this neuromuscular disorder, and these continue to be studied.

Although there is no known cure for cerebral palsy, early and aggressive treatment can allow for children and adults with the disorder to experience full and functional lives with minimal disadvantage. Early recognition allows for optimal utilization of physical therapy services. Speech and occupational therapy are also utilized. Assistive devices such as braces, wheel chairs, walkers, and braces are available options. In some cases, surgery may be required to release tight muscles. Additionally, medications for pain and muscle spasm may be utilized. Cerebral palsy may also affect the muscles that allow for clear speech and communication; therefore, alternative communication devices may be offered. Goals of therapy should aim to maximize independent functioning.

Hip dysplasia in children

Developmental dysplasia of the hip (DDH) is possible in any newborn. However, there certain trends have been noted. DDH does appear to run in families. It seems to affect the left hip more frequently than the right. Females and first-borns are more susceptible. Breech birthing position also increases the risk. Along with positive Ortolani's and Barlow's signs, several asymmetries can be noted with mere visualization in the infant with DDH. Leg length will be unequal, shorter on the affected side. Posterior skin fold of in the gluteal and thigh region will be asymmetric. Decreased use and movement of the dysplastic hip may be noted. In the older patient, the gait will appear more like a waddle.

Early detection of developmental dysplasia of the hip (DDH) is important for noninvasive treatment and best long-term prognosis. If DDH is diagnosed in a newborn, and closed reduction maneuvers do not maintain hip location, a Pavlik harness is often utilized for a few months. If this is unsuccessful, or in the case of later diagnosis, closed reduction with anesthesia may be performed, followed by placement of a cast. This is the common method up to 2 years of age. DDH that persist or is not diagnosed beyond two year of age require open surgical reduction followed by placement of body spica cast.

Ortolani's sign and Barlow's sign

Ortolani's sign: this test is used to check for a dislocated hip(s) in an infant. The examiners thumb is placed on the distal and medial femur and the other four fingers are at the proximal head of the femur (maintaining upward pressure with fingers). The infants' hip and knee are flexed at 90 degrees and slowly abducted. A positive Ortolani's sign will result in a pop, which is a relocation of a dislocated hip.
Barlow's sign: this test assess' infant hip stability. The infant will be supine with hips and knees flexed at 90 degrees and hips abducted. Examining position will be the same as in the Ortolani's test, with the exception of a downward pressure of the four fingers on the femoral head. Slow adduction will result in palpable shift as the head of the femur dislocates from its socket. This results in a positive Barlow's sign.

Pavlik harness

The Pavlik harness is commonly used in the first few months of life when an infant is diagnosed with developmental hip dysplasia. This is a sort splint device that maintains the hips and knees at 90 degrees while the hips are fully abducted. It is important to show the parents, using a model, that this position is necessary in maintaining the let in the hip socket. This is a natural and comfortable position for the newborn, and parents should not be alarmed by it, or worry that it is hurting their child. Parents should be instructed on proper placement can care of the splint. They should be taught and then observed in correct technique of dressing, bathing, diapering, holding, transferring and positioning of the infant with this brace. Skin care should be thoroughly reviewed.

Pes cavus

Pes cavus is used to describe an abnormally elevated foot arch. It is sometimes called "clawfoot". If this is seen in children under six years of age, suspect (or at least rule-out) a neuromuscular disorder, as this is a rare finding in children. Eliminate muscle spasm or weakness and spinal etiology as the cause of elevated arches. As the child grows, parents may not difficulty fitting shoes and frequent ankle sprains. Pain is only a complaint of pes cavus later in life. Orthotics and arch supports are the primary treatment in childhood.

Congenital torticollis

Congenital muscular torticollis is caused by a constant unilateral contraction or tightness in the sternocleidomastoid muscle of the neck. Shortening this muscle results in lateral flexion of the head to that side. At the same time, the chin is simultaneously pointed slightly to the opposite side, and off of midline. Parents either note lack of head movement to one side or are alarmed by a "knot" that is felt along the proximal attachment site of the tightened muscle on the sternum. This knot disappears with treatment and resolution of the condition. Treatment is primarily conservative with physical therapy, massage, bracing and positioning. A significant proportion of infants born with torticollis will also have hip dysplasia.

"Pigeon toe"

In-toeing and pigeon toed are terms used interchangeably to describe a common childhood anomaly. Pigeon toes are not a disorder of the feet at all. Under the age of 2, this gait or stance is usually secondary to a slightly rotated tibial bone. This gait is usually self-limited and does not require treatment. In the child over age 3, in-toeing may signify twisting of the femur. This is not self-limiting. Bracing and physical therapy have not proven effective. Surgery is only indicated if this condition causes pain, disability or significant leg asymmetry.

Talipes equinovarus

Talipes equinovarus is more commonly termed 'clubfoot'. Clubfoot is a fairly common birth deformity that can be unilateral or bilateral, and is usually easily detected. The foot is positioned abnormally in three directions. First the heel points medially and is inverted. Second, the ankle points in the inferior direction. Third, the entire foot appears supinated (plantar surface up). If this is detected in a newborn, maintain a high index of suspicion for neuromuscular disease and hip dysplasia. Treatment is primarily manual manipulation followed by splinting or casting with frequent follow-up and gradual anatomical repositioning. Prognosis is good with early treatment. Complications or lack-of treatment can result in long-term disability and deformity.

Congenital limb absence

Congenital absence of the arm and leg (at various levels), and the thumb are possible but infrequent. When a child is born without a limb, several factors in management need to be considered. After assuring the health and stabilization of the newborn, including careful evaluation of the major organ systems, much of the care involves the parents. The parents will need a variety of counseling, education and support. Medical specialty evaluation (especially orthopedic) is necessary to further reassure the parents, and alleviate anxiety. Speaking to different medical specialties, allows the parents to understand and adjust to their child's birth defect. Reconstruction and prosthetics are rarely considered or necessary before 2 years of age. Function and patient self-image issues should outweigh surgical risks and parent insecurities when evaluating surgical and/or prosthetic options.

Bowlegs and knock-knees

Bowlegs are termed 'genu varum'. Genu varum is an anomaly in which the tibia and fibula are angled medially in relation to the femur. This is a common finding under the age of 2. Bowlegs usually resolve themselves, if not, bracing has been successful into the third decade. Surgery is only indicated if genu varum affects growth or is asymmetrical. Genu valgum is the medical term used to describe knock-knees. The lower leg is laterally deviated compared to the upper leg in this disorder. Knock-knees are usually seen after 3 years of age, after resolution of bowlegs. Lateral deviation of the lower leg can be considered normal beyond 10 degrees of deviation. Genu valgum is often outgrown and does not respond to shoe inserts or braces. Monitor growth and reassure parents with both of these conditions.

Limb length discrepancies

Limb length discrepancies (LLD) occur for a number of reasons and many people have some amount of asymmetry in length. However, treatment is only a consideration in those with greater than 1 inch discrepancy and if it causes significant gait disturbance and pain, especially in the back. Shoe lifts are the initial treatment choice. These are inexpensive and can be modified. Leg-shortening surgical procedures are primarily options for the skeletally immature. Results are not immediate, and a complication is miscalculation of bone growth resulting in uneven limbs in the opposite direction. Leg-lengthening procedures are for the skeletally mature, reliable and compliant patient. This is a lengthy process and involves close monitoring and frequent follow-up. Infection risk is greater than limb-shortening procedures, due to the external fixator that is used.

Legg-Calve-Perthes disease

Legg-Calve-Perthes (LCP) disease is a disorder in which the head of the femur deteriorates due to temporary lack of blood supply. It affects more males than females, ages 3-9. Other risk factors include: race, low-birth weight, short-stature, second-hand smoke exposure, and first-born children. It is more often unilateral. It is self-limiting, but bracing, pain management, and physical therapy are important for a good prognosis. Patient/parent education focusing on the typical disease progression and healing timeline are paramount. Complications of noncompliance or inadequate treatment are deformity, decreased range of motion, and early-onset osteoarthritis.

Myelomeningocele

Patient with the most severe form of spina bifida require a multi-medical team approach as well as patient and caregiver education. Early deformities that may be evident in this patient type largely involve the lower extremities. Foot deformities such as talipes equinovarus, calcaneus and cavus are common. Hip dysplasia is also common. Muscle atrophy and loss of bone density will be seen in extremities below the level of spinal cord involvement. Contractures abnormal spinal curvatures are also an orthopedic concern in the patient with spina bifida. Appropriate treatment and management, of the above conditions, must be implemented.

Spina bifida

Spina bifida is a congenital disorder in which the development of the brain and/or spinal cord and its covering is abnormal. There are four types of spina bifida. From most common and mild spina bifida to its most severe forms are: occulta, closed-neural tube defect, meningocele, and myelomeningocele. Often times the nondescript term 'spina bifida' is synonymously used with the term to describe the most severe form of the disease, 'myelomeningocele'. The first three types of spina bifida may go undiagnosed and have few or no neurologic deficits. The fourth and most severe type of spina bifida (myelomeningocele) will result in the external exposure of the spinal cord, resulting in paralysis below the level of exposure. There is often multi-organ dysfunction in this case.

Salter-Harris classification system

The Salter-Harris classification system is used to describe a child's fracture and its involvement with the growth plate (physis). This system has 5 stages numbered using Roman numerals. Type I is a fracture through the growth plate itself, increasing the width of the physis and not disrupting the epiphysis or metaphysis. Type II fractures are through the physis and metaphysis, not involving the epiphysis. This is the most common fracture. Type III involves a fracture through the physis and epiphysis. Type IV fractures pass vertically through the epiphysis, physis and metaphysis. Finally, Salter-Harris Type V fractures completely compress of crush the physis with no fracture of the epiphysis or metaphysis.

Osteogenesis imperfecta

Osteogenesis imperfecta (OI) is commonly known as "brittle bone disease". This is hereditary and a child may be born with multiple fractures or sustain fractures frequently with activities that would not normally cause a bone to break. There are four types of OI, based on severity. Treatment focuses on prevention, developing and maintaining bone mass, working on muscle strength, and minimizing complications. Acute management involves appropriate reduction and immobilization. Review cast care. Pain management options include: ice, heat, TENS unit, medication and nerve blocks. Chronic treatment and prevention includes: appropriate low-impact exercise, physical therapy, and nutrition counseling.

Scoliosis

Scoliosis is often seen in children during routine examinations, whether they have complaints of pain or not. Simple observation of body symmetry can lead to the diagnosis of scoliosis. It is best to examine the patient with as few clothing obstructions as possible. Examine them from the front and back, standing, walking and with forward flexion at the waist. The patient with scoliosis will often display asymmetrical shoulder blades, iliac crests and waist creases. X-rays will confirm diagnosis and establish quantitative measurement. Observation is recommended in the child with less than 20 degrees of curvature. Consider back brace with up to 40 degrees of curvature and complaint of back pain, disfigurement and gait impairment. A child with greater than 40 degrees of curvature is a surgical candidate.

Amputees concerns in children

Child amputees often have a much smaller learning curve than adults. Not only does the stump heal quicker and with less pain, but also stump end-point or maturation is rapid. This allows for earlier fitting of prosthetic limbs, with fewer adjustments. The child with lower limb amputation begins walking rapidly with a prosthetic limb. However, ease of use of an upper extremity prosthetic may take more time for a child to master versus an adult. A child amputee will rarely experience phantom limb pains. A complication unique to childhood amputations is the high rate of bony overgrowth, which often results in multiple stump revisions.

Inflammatory Disorders

Rheumatoid arthritis

Rheumatoid arthritis (RA) is genetic autoimmune disease. It is a disorder in which the body's own immune system turns on itself and starts to attack itself. RA can affect any body system but is most often initially discovered when a patient complains of persistent joint pain. In the case of joint disease in RA, the body attacks the synovium of the joint, which causes swelling, and thickening of this area. The damage often extends to the surrounding joint structures including bone. RA can be progressive or be marked by the exacerbation and remission cycle. The hands, wrists, shoulders, knees, and feet are most often affected, usually bilaterally.

Management of the patient with rheumatoid arthritis (RA) is a multisystem approach. Controlling pain and maintaining function are the goals of management. These goals are accomplished by medications and clear instruction on their purpose, uses, side effects and monitoring. Assuring compliance with medications promotes remission of the RA. Patient education regarding the compromised state of their immune system is important so they can take steps to reduce anything preventable that would further compromise them. The importance of regular sleep and exercise, good nutrition, proper body mechanics, use of assistive devices and regular flu shots are important in maintaining the health of their immune system. Psychological health and counseling should be addressed including their support systems. Activities of daily living including self-care, occupational and hobbies should all be assessed to avoid undue stress on the joints. Patient should not be lost to follow up.

The cornerstones for treatment of rheumatoid arthritis (RA) are the class of drugs called: disease-modifying anti-rheumatic drugs (DMARDs). These medications actually slow the progression and joint deformities of the disease. They also encourage remission. For acute exacerbations analgesics, nonsteroidal anti-inflammatories, COX-2 inhibitors, and corticosteroids may be used. The antimalarial drug Plaquenil has been effective in modifying the course of RA. Immunomodulators are also a treatment option; these help prevent the structural joint damage that occurs with RA. A newer class of medications combating RA is the biologic response modifiers; these are injectable and intravenous only. All classes of medications are often used in various combinations for the best disease control. These medications all have significant side effects and require thorough patient education and monitoring.

Juvenile rheumatoid arthritis (JRA) and its 3 subtypes

JRA is an autoimmune disease similar to rheumatoid arthritis except that it affects patients under 16 years of age. Prognosis is good, as most children will "grow-out" of this disease. However, joint damage sustained in the childhood disease will always be present, even though the progressive disease ends. The most common subtype of JRA is polyarticular onset. This involves greater than 5 joints, unilateral or bilateral, and is often severe and sudden in its onset. Children with this subtype are at increased risk for permanent joint deformity. Pauciarticular onset is the second most common type of JRA. This subtype does not affect more than 4 joints. Pauciarticular JRA more often affects the joints of the lower extremities. A major complication of a patient that develops this form of JRA before age 6 is chronic eye disease and complications. Finally, systemic onset JRA is the third subtype. This is diagnosed in a patient with recurring spiking fevers and truncal rash in addition to their joint pains. A rare complication of this type of JRA is pericarditis.

The first nursing challenge associated with JRA may be obtaining a history and progress report from the parent or child. The younger the child, the less likely they will be able to describe their symptoms. Care must be taken in obtaining a history from the parents and questions should be specific to the child's daily activities. In addition to managing JRA with medications, therapy and splinting, the emotional well-being must be nurtured. Every effort to maintain self-esteem and optimal school participation must be made. All close contacts (family, siblings, teachers) should be educated on the child with JRA and ways to modify activities in an inclusive versus exclusive manner.

RA vs. SLE

Both RA (rheumatoid arthritis) and SLE (systemic lupus erythematosus) are autoimmune disorders that affect a greater percentage of females. It is theorized that both have a genetic component. Although, both SLE and RA can affect all body systems, the musculoskeletal system is primarily affected in RA. Both disease states primarily have a bilateral distribution of joint symptoms. Typically in SLE, the distal joints are most often affected. RA affects distal joints as well as hips, knees and shoulders located more proximally. Both cause morning stiffness and may result in inflamed joints. Disability of the musculoskeletal system is usually greater in RA than SLE. The age of onset is earlier for SLE than RA. Treatment and disease management are similar for both including prescription medication options. Management with physical therapy, joint protection, assistive devices, nutritional counseling and psychological counseling are important for both disease states.

Systemic lupus erythematosus (SLE)

The orthopedic evaluation of a patient with SLE should not be limited to the musculoskeletal system. Although SLE can affect all body systems, often times it is the visible skin changes that bring them in for evaluation. Characteristic skin findings can give a clue to the diagnosis; long before joint and muscle signs may be appreciated. Classic skin finding of SLE include: butterfly rash over the cheeks, discoid lesions, vascular changes in the digits, and erythematous plaques. If skin conditions appear after sun exposure, suspect SLE. Splinter hemorrhages may appear in the nail/nail bed and thinning of scalp hair are other findings. Exam of muscle and joints includes decreased mobility, redness, and diffuse swelling. Joint findings are secondary to inflammation of the joint synovium and fibrous tissue replacing muscle. Jaccoud's deformity may be noted which is evidenced by ulnar deviation of the MCP joints and hyperextension of the PIP joints of the hand.

Polymyositis

Polymyositis, also termed idiopathic inflammatory myopathy, refers to a disease that affects muscle fibers and connective tissue. It is chronic with exacerbation and remissions. Polymyositis can affect the entire body, but effects on the musculoskeletal system are most common and more evident. The immune system attack the muscle, causing chronic swelling of muscle fibers, this leads to muscle weakness and eventual atrophy. The proximal muscle groups are the most commonly affected, including the hips and shoulders, usually symmetrically. The cause of polymyositis is unknown. It is more common in females. Diagnosis includes history of muscle weakness, blood work including creatine kinase levels, EMG testing and biopsy. Treatment is primarily with oral corticosteroids. Complications of polymyositis include neck muscle weakness causing swallowing difficulties and difficulty breathing if it affects the muscles of the chest. Complications of treatment with long-term corticosteroid are the development of diabetes, osteoporosis and skin changes.

Ankylosing spondylitis

Ankylosing spondylitis (AS) is an inflammatory disorder primarily affecting the disc spaces, costovertebral joints and the sacroiliac joint. AS causes these joints can become fused over time. AS does not affect joints symmetrically and the RF blood test is negative. A patient with AS will not develop nodular formations over their joints, and they are more likely to be a young male of average age 25. The synovium of the joint is not affected; rather, the site where ligament attaches to bone is affected. Comorbidities of AS include: arthritis of the large joints, uveitis, Crohn's disease-like symptoms, fibrotic lungs, and aortic insufficiency all of which shorten the life expectancy.

Early stages of AS may not reveal many physical exam findings. There are 3 important objective tests that, if positive, suggest the diagnosis of AS. First, the Wright-Schober test is positive if lumbar spine flexion is < 5 cm. marking the L5-S1 level and 10 cm above this level on a standing patient measure this. Forward flexion in a healthy person, increases the distance between the 2 markers by at least 5 cm. Second, the respiratory excursion tests measures the resting distance between the nipples, this test is positive for AS if the measurement does not increase by at least 3 cm with full inspiration. Third, measurement of cervical kyphosis is positive for AS if patient cannot touch the back of their head to the wall when their heels and entire posterior body is against the wall. This test can also be utilized to monitor progression of AS.

Bursitis

There are over 100 bursa in the body that serve as a cushion between tendon and bone by lubricating the area with synovial fluid. The most commonly spoke-of bursa disorders occur at the shoulder, elbow, hip and knee. With repetitive us of these joints, the bursa can become inflamed and painful.

Bursitis can also develop secondary to trauma, infection, gout, and a sudden increase in activity level such as in 'weekend warriors'. This condition can be acute or chronic. Self-care should be aimed at preventing chronicity with advice in proper stretching, warm-up and body mechanics. Management of acute bursitis is with RICE therapy and anti-inflammatories. Rarely are invasive treatments indicated, these would include aspiration of bursa, injection with steroid, or complete removal of the bursa.

Psoriatic arthritis treatment options

Psoriatic arthritis can be managed with patient education and involvement. Stretching should be regular to reduce the likelihood of contracture and joint stress. Determination of exercise tolerance and rest and recovery period should be established. Appropriate footwear should be emphasized. Topical treatment of psoriasis skin lesions may result in a combination of agents with or without ultraviolet A light therapy. Anti-inflammatories, aspirin, DMARDs, biological modifiers, and steroids may all be helpful as they are also recommended for rheumatoid arthritis. Use precaution with anti-inflammatories, as this may flare the psoriatic skin conditions. Alternative therapies include: sea salts, massage, acupuncture, meditation, glucosamine, SAM-e, and magnet therapy.

Systemic sclerosis

Systemic sclerosis can affect all body systems. Its affect on the musculoskeletal system extends from bones and muscles to joints and tendons. In terms of the affect on bone, it softens the bone causing reabsorption and eventual atrophy of bone structure. The comorbidity associated with this is osteoporosis. The bones most affected are those of the distal upper extremity, jawbone and ribs. Muscle is replaced with inelastic fibrous tissue. Joint synovium also becomes fibrotic leading to multiple joint pains and restrictions. The tendons are affected similarly as fibrous deposits develop here, causing swelling and restriction of smooth movement of tendon over joints. Carpal tunnel syndrome is also likely to develop as a complication of systemic sclerosis on the tendons.

Scleroderma

Scleroderma is a rheumatic disease in which the skin and connective tissue, throughout the body, becomes fibrotic, hardened and tight. This happens to excess collagen production. The thickening action of the skin and tissue creates an appearance of the skin being shiny and 'pulled-tight' over bone. This is especially apparent over joints. This tension and loss of skin elasticity creates a wrinkle-free appearance and pigmentation can also change in these areas. Increased incidence of scleroderma is seen in females, black females, and increasingly after age 40. The cause of scleroderma is unknown.

Important Terms

Swan-neck deformity: this is a common deformity of the fingers seen in the autoimmune disease of rheumatoid arthritis. The deformity is caused by damage to the synovium placing the DIP and MCP joints in flexion, while the PIP joint of the affected digit is hyperextended. Management options include various splints, disease modifying anti-rheumatic drugs, or surgical options that usually involve tendon release.

Boutonniere deformity: this is a deformity of the finger(s) usually seen in rheumatoid arthritis, but it can also be present after "jamming the finger". The deformity involves damage to the extensor tendons leading to hyperextension of the DIP joint and flexion of the PIP joint. Treatment includes nonsteroidal anti-inflammatory drugs, disease modifying anti-rheumatic drugs, splinting, occupational therapy, and surgery only as a last resort.

Polymyositis: causes muscle inflammation, weakness and atrophy of truncal muscle groups. It is twice as common in females and tends to first be seen in the teens and around 50 years of age.

Dermatomyositis: similar to polymyositis with additional affect on the skin tissue, causing widespread skin rash and changes including permanent bumps underneath the skin. It is more common in women and associated with increased risk of malignancy, especially ovarian cancer.

Inclusion body myositis: causes widespread muscle weakness in atrophy, predominately in the distal muscle groups. It can also cause difficulties with swallowing like polymyositis can. This form of myositis is more common in males and after age 50. There are no effective medication treatment options for this type.

Juvenile myositis: this is a combination of the above myopathies found in the pediatric patient. They often go on to develop the characteristic skin changes of dermatomyositis.

Operative Orthopaedics

Blood loss from orthopedic surgery

Assessment: A patient may display several signs and symptoms that suggest blood loss/volume depletion. Many of these signs and symptoms can be seen in other conditions as well. Maintain a high index of suspicion. Visually assess patient for any external signs of blood loss, including checking bandages. Do not forget universal precautions while doing this. Vague symptoms of blood loss can include vertigo, fatigue and anxious feelings, also seen with pain medications. Patient may also complain of pain and weakness. Vitals would demonstrate tachypnea, low blood pressure, and rapid heart rate. Patient will also likely be diaphoretic. Any of these signs should prompt lab work. Management: Secondly, the source of bleeding must be determined and the bleeding stopped. There are several methods to decrease loss of blood, from simple pressure application to electrocauterization. If hemoglobin levels less than 6 g/dL, transfusion is likely.

Major types of anesthesia

There are three major types of anesthesia:

- General Anesthesia: it is important that nursing staff is available when the patient is "going under" and "coming out of" the anesthesia. The nurse may assist with intubation and evaluating its placement. It is also important to assist with vitals, return of mental state, reflexes, and check for any side effects anesthesia may have caused.
- Regional Anesthesia: primarily staying alert for all signs and symptoms of allergic reaction by monitoring vitals and nervous system complaints or signs. Assess return of function to anesthetized area.

- Conscious Sedation + Local: patient is able to verbally respond to your monitoring of their pain and comfort levels. Assess vitals.

Possible signs and symptoms of postoperative pulmonary embolism

The post surgical patient may complain of sudden shortness of breath, pain with inspiration, chest pain and cough. You may find them to be slightly tachycardic, have a decreased oxygen saturation, appear slightly anxious and with rapid breaths or the occasional attempt at a deep inspiration (they often appear to be hyperventilating). Lung sounds, blood pressure, chest x-ray and EKG may all be within normal limits, especially in early stages. Maintain a high index of suspicion, as this is the major post surgical complication, especially with total joint replacement procedures.

If pulmonary embolism is suspected, the next important step is obtaining tests to help confirm this. D-dimer is a good blood test, but in the post operative setting it may display a greater number of false-positives. The V/Q (ventilation/perfusion) lung scan is still considered the gold standard for diagnosis of pulmonary embolism. However, the CT angiogram is becoming more widely used with similar accuracy. Determining which test to use depends on a number of factors, but availability and accessibility should be of primary concern. One of these imaging studies should be ordered and performed in a timely manner, as delay in diagnosis and thus treatment, could be fatal.

The nurse's role in such a situation is vital, and includes assuring stabilization of all vitals, including oxygen if needed. Initially, rest is important with frequent non-weight bearing range of motion exercises while in bed. After stabilization is reached, add in weight bearing activities as tolerated. Maintain regular diet and hydration. As patient will be on IV heparin and then coumadin, frequent PTT/INR (partial thromboplastin time/international normalized ratio) must be drawn. Thorough patient education with discharge instructions regarding the numerous side effects and drug and food interactions of the coumadin (warfarin) is an absolute must. Patients also need to be instructed on the frequent monitoring of this medication, with frequent blood draws and monitoring to keep INR in the 2.0: 3.0 range. Therapy and monitoring will continue for at least 3 months. If the patient is female and of childbearing age, you need to instruct her on finding a non-estrogenic contraceptive method.

Compartment syndrome

Compartment syndrome is a condition in which an area of the body accumulates an increased amount of pressure within the muscle, causing damage to surrounding tissue. There are several compartments in the body, and those most commonly affected are in the extremities. A compartment is an anatomical site that contains muscle, arteries, veins, nerves and bone surrounded by fascia. Fascia is not all that flexible, so when there is increased volume or swelling within the compartment that creates dangerous pressure levels. The increased pressure cuts off nerve and vessel circulation to the muscle, if uncorrected muscle death occurs rapidly. Causes of increased compartmental pressure can be external or internal. There are 3 types of compartment syndrome. There are several compartments within the leg and this is the most common site for the syndrome to occur.

Acute compartment syndrome is a medical emergency. Without rapid intervention loss of limb and even loss of life can occur. With an increased pressure gradient, vasculature structures within the compartment collapse. This prevents delivery of oxygen and nutrients to the muscle, nerve and bone causing necrosis. Causes of acute compartment syndrome are: deeply bruised muscle or a surgical complication. The injury usually occurs proximal to the compartment affected, cutting off circulation to all compartments distally.

Examination findings will include change in skin color, sensation, temperature and pulse distal to the area of trauma. Passive range of elongation of affected muscle groups will reproduce pain.

Rapid recognition and action is the key to successful outcome. The cause of increased compartment pressure needs to be identified and removed. If external devices are the cause, they need removed, repositioned or loosened. Examples of external pressure may be automatic blood pressure cuff monitors, casts, braces, compression stockings, or incorrect positioning. Limb elevation is not recommended; the limb should remain at heart level. Debridment is recommended for acute compartment syndrome secondary to burn victims. Fasciotomy is definitive and often still necessary after removing external pressure sources. Fasciotomy is indicated when compartment pressures are >30 mm HG and when clinical findings are present. Delayed closure is used after fasciotomy, usually at least 3 days after the procedure.

Crush compartment syndrome

Crush compartment syndrome is damage to a body compartment from an external source. Injury at the bony level causes bleeding and swelling that can create increased compartmental pressure and rapid muscle necrosis. Damaged muscle tissue releases myoglobin. These increased levels of myoglobin can rapidly overwhelm the kidneys. Therefore, not only will the patient complain of pain and swelling, but also there will likely be systemic manifestations. Examples are: an extremity being lodged underneath a heavy object such as a car, falling asleep with a limb in a position that cuts of circulation, and external medical equipment (casts, traction, incorrect surgical positions, and surgical closure of fascial injury).

Chronic compartment syndrome

Chronic compartment syndrome is not a medical emergency. A frequent and high level of exercise causes it. The compartmental pressure builds during physical activity, causing pain. It is rapidly relieved by cessation of exercise, even though above-normal compartment pressures may remain. Chronic compartment syndrome most commonly affects the legs of runners. In addition to pain, they may have difficulty with foot movements. Swelling is usually minimal and compartment involvement is often bilateral. Conservative treatment includes physical therapy, avoiding or altering triggers, orthotics, anti-inflammatories, and diuretics. If these measures fail, definitive treatment with surgical fasciotomy is indicated.

Preoperative surgical considerations

Preoperative planning and tasks are important for the overall surgical outcome. Obtain a thorough history of the operative patient with emphasis on medication and latex allergies. Assess their current medications for anesthetic and pain medication interactions and to properly recommend the interval for presurgical discontinuation. Review family health history and social history for evaluation of postsurgical support. Physical exam includes recording all vitals including height and weight. Determine if there are current signs of infection, and follow with appropriate action. For intubation and airway access concerns, note the dentation of the patient, neck extension ability and open mouth space. Obtain lab studies and informed consent. Thorough patient education is also necessary.

Fat embolism syndrome

Fat embolism syndrome (FES) is seen with traumatic long bone fracture. Risk for FES increases is there are multiple long bone fractures or pelvic bone fractures. Fat emboli are released into circulation after bony trauma or surgical procedure. Initial signs of fat emboli are respiratory changes and difficulty, mental status changes, skin changes and thrombocytopenia. The diagnosis of FES is primarily clinical and a diagnosis of exclusion. A high index of suspicion should exist with marked hypoxemia and arterial blood gas and other lab work changes resulting in metabolic acidosis. Treatment is supportive and is aimed at normalizing the metabolic acidosis, restoring volume and maintaining respiratory function.

Intraoperative complications

Cardiovascular: operative ischemia and myocardial infarction are causes of surgical mortality. Use of opioids, oxygen and inhalation agents can decrease the stress on the heart muscle and increase oxygen available. Preoperative history should identify patients that are at high risk for this complication. Pulmonary: the most common complication of the lungs in surgery is aspiration. Treatment of this includes maintaining the airway, suctioning and oxygen. Prevention lies largely on compliance of the preoperative fast. Hypovolemia: surgical blood loss is probable, however, careful monitoring and surgical technique can keep blood loss to a minimum. Complications occur when there is significant volume depletion. Bleeding site must be located, bleeding controlled, and replacement given if necessary. Prevention of bleeding depends on compliance of discontinuation of preoperative aspirin and anti-inflammatory medication.

Preoperative patient education

Patient teachings and knowledge of the upcoming procedure are key components of successful outcome. Much of the educating process should take place in the early preoperative phase or several days before surgery. This allows plenty of time for patients to process, have their questioned answers, and inform you of possible important history facts that they may have deemed unimportant or irrelevant initially. Successful patient education will result in absent to minimized surgical anxiety. Inform patient with written instructions on preoperative fast, medicine discontinuation, and smoking cessation. Discuss the reasons for this and complications so they are more likely to comply. Review safety precautions and calling for help. Review presurgical procedures such as IV access, catheterization and oxygen. Finally, educate the patient on postoperative expectations for pain (and management) and rehabilitation.

Virchow's triad

Virchow's triad is a term to describe 3 conditions that contribute to the formation of deep vein thrombosis (DVT). The first condition is vessel wall damage. The second condition is the decreased rate of blood flow. The third component of the triad is increased blood clotting. DVT's are a common complication following total hip and knee replacements. Increased operative risks for DVT are: incorrect surgical positioning, use of proximal tourniquets, and excessive surgical movement of the limb. Other risk factors for DVT include: age, comorbidities, smoking, use of hormones, clotting disorders, fractures, and prolonged immobilization. Prevention includes correction of risk factors and medicinal and mechanical surgical prophylaxis.

Temperature regulation

Low body temperature or hypothermia is a surgical complication in which the body temperature drops below 96.8 degrees. This is more common at patients at both age extremes and with surgery of the proximal body cavities. Hypothermia increases the risk of infection, bleeding, heart problems, and delayed healing. Prevention includes: constant temperature monitoring, warming IV fluids, increasing room temperature, and use of blankets. On the other hand, increased surgical body temperature (malignant hyperthermia) is a life-threatening emergency. Patients inherit this trait and it becomes life threatening at temperatures greater than 110 degrees Fahrenheit. Many anesthetic agents can trigger this response. Early signs of hyperthermia are rigidity, increased arterial carbon dioxide, and increased respirations and heart rate. Cardiac arrest follows without rapid treatment and reversal. Reversal and normalization of body temperature includes discontinuation of offending agents, oxygen, IV dantrolene, and external cooling devices and techniques.

Metabolic Bone Disease

Osteoporosis

Osteoporosis is a skeletal disorder in which the density of the bone is decreased. This happens as a result of increased bone resorption (increased osteoclast activity) and decreased bone formation (decreased osteoblast activity). This results in decreased strength of bone and increased likelihood of bony fractures. It is the most common metabolic bone disease. It is more common after 50 years of age and in women. White and Asian women are at increased risk. Smokers and patients that consume large amounts of caffeine and alcohol increase their risk for osteoporosis. Those with low body fat and weight and a small frame are at increased risk, this is often seen in females with eating disorders and female marathon runners. There appears to be a genetic component in the development of osteoporosis. Chronic use of steroid medications, excess/inappropriate amounts of thyroid medication, and decreased weight bearing activity increases the risks for osteoporosis.

Goals of treatment for osteoporosis are fracture reduction, maintenance of skeletal strength and function, and pain reduction. Recommend regular weight bearing exercise, smoking cessation, and discontinuation or reduction in caffeine and alcohol for all. Increased dietary or supplementary calcium intake is indicated in almost all cases. Recommended amounts of Vitamin D should be taken in conjunction with and calcium supplementation. Prescription medication options also include: hormone replacement, calcitonin (injection or nasal), bisphosphanates (Fosamax and Actonel), fluoride, and Evista. Some of these may be used in combination, and patient selection is important.

Often-times osteoporosis is an incidental finding after a fracture. X-ray films may show the initial decreased bone density. Osteoporosis should also be suspected when a fall minor fall or injury results in a fracture. Other signs of the disease are decreased height measurements at the annual physical exam and increase thoracic kyphosis. These findings are a result of vertebral lose of height and compression fracture. The gold standard for osteoporosis diagnosis is the DEXA scan, which measure BMD (bone mineral density). Typically this is measured at the hip and spine. Measures less than 2.5 SD indicate osteoporosis. Lab work should be obtained to rule out other causes of osteoporosis.

Vitamin nutrients

Calcium: is important for all components of bone health. Although this is a common supplement, plenty of food sources contain rich amounts of calcium. Dairy products and dark green, vegetables contain the most natural calcium. Appropriate levels of Vitamin D must also be present for calcium to be absorbed and utilized; otherwise the calcium will just be excreted through the urine.
Vitamin D: as stated above, this helps with the body's absorption calcium. Many foods that contain adequate Vitamin D, are also high in fat (butter, eggs, cheese, and fatty fish). Therefore, the best way for a patient to obtain adequate Vitamin D, besides supplementation, is with safe exposure to sunlight.
Magnesium: about 50% of the body's magnesium is found in bone. Dietary sources of magnesium include: meat and fish, fruits, grains, and nuts.
Phosphate: this is helpful in bone metabolism. Good dietary sources of phosphate are dairy products and meat.

Prevention measures

Prevention measures in the elderly person may imply disease prevention, disease progression, or disease complication. Supplementation and nutritional counseling are primary. Include regular weight bearing activity. Reduce or eliminate smoking, alcohol, and caffeine. Reducing the risk of falls in this age group is probably the most important. This age group is at increased risk of falls secondary to visual changes, mobility and strength changes, dementia, increased toileting needs, and medication side effects. Reducing risk of falls, and thus fractures, includes review of medications and evaluation of living environment. Creating easier and unobstructed paths within the house is important. Remove throw rugs, rearrange furniture, limit use of stairs, and create adequate lighting with use of motion lights and nightlights. Assistive devices are helpful if the patient is trained in the proper use.

Prevention and patient education regarding the development of osteoporosis in the younger patient differs slightly from the education of an elderly patient. Patient education should start in the late teens and should be reinforced throughout the twenties. This is because maximal bone density and mass is achieved at about 20 year of age, after that there is a natural decline. Education should be aimed at preventing and slowing this decline. Education for the younger age group emphasizes a healthy weight through nutrition and exercise. Nutrition and caloric intake is especially important in the endurance athlete and those that participate in sports that require a certain body type and size such as dancing and gymnastics. Osteoporosis is one of the complications of eating disorders as well. Educate the patient that develops amenorrhea or has an early surgical menopause, on their risks for developing osteoporosis.

Gout

Gout is a term used to define a number of metabolic bone disorders that result in either over-production or under-secretion of uric acid. This results in the accumulation of uric acid within the joint. This causes pain, swelling, redness and warmth over the affected joint. Over time, uric acid crystals can replace bone. Males are at increased risk for the development of gout. Other risk factors include: obesity, hyperlipidemia, excess alcohol consumption, and increased dietary consumption of red meat, sardines, and liver. Several medications have also been implicated in the development of gout including: diuretics, low-dose aspirin, B-complex vitamins, and many chemotherapy drugs.

Treatment of gout primarily centers on medications. However, nutritional counseling and prevention is still important. Medication options range from acute treatment and chronic maintenance or preventative therapy. Usually these are used in combination. Common prophylactic drugs include: colchicines, probenecid and allopurinol. Indomethacin is an anti-inflammatory most commonly used to treat acute attacks. Like all anti-inflammatories, indomethacin can cause varying levels of gastritis. Use it with caution in appropriate patients, stressing the importance of taking it with food and signs and symptoms of concern. Patient tolerability to these medications is sometimes difficult, and it may take time and trial of different combinations before finding the optimal individualized therapy. If inadequate treatments, over time bone destruction, kidney disease and tophi can occur.

Osteitis deformans

Osteitis deformans is better known as Paget's disease. It is a metabolic bone disorder in which there is increased bone breakdown. The body compensates for this by rapid bone remodeling. This results in bones appearing larger, but they are in fact, structurally weaker. These structurally modified bones are at risk for fracture and deformity, causing the patient with Paget's disease pain. The areas most commonly affected are bones of the skull, spine, pelvis and legs. The cause of Paget's disease is unknown and treatment is supportive. Treatment cannot reverse the disease, but can stabilize it and reduce pain. Treatment options include physical and thermotherapy, stretching and medications. Maintenance medications include those from the bisphosphonate class and acute treatment is with anti-inflammatories and analgesics.

Osteomalacia and osteoporosis

Osteomalacia is a decrease in the mineral composition of the bone, causing softening of the bone. This is primarily due to decreased Vitamin D. Osteoporosis is decreased density and mass of bone, largely secondarily to decreased Calcium. Both conditions present with complaints of bone pain, muscle pain, and fractures. Causes of osteomalacia are: dysfunctional Vitamin D absorption, decreased sunlight exposure, and medications such as seizure drugs and fluoride. Osteoporosis is caused by age, lack of hormone and calcium, and drugs such as anti-inflammatories.

Osteomalacia can be reversed and treated, osteoporosis can only be stabilized but not reversed.

Hypoparathyroidism

Hypoparathyroidism is a condition in which the parathyroid glands secret too little parathyroid hormone. This can happen for a number of reasons: genetic, alcoholism, injury to gland in surgery, GI surgeries that result in malabsorption, GI disorders, and liver and pancreas disease.

Hypoparathyroidism is marked by hypocalcemia, and the affects of this on the body. Musculoskeletal findings from the hypocalcemia of hypoparathyroidism include vague pain symptoms, anxiety, muscle rigidity, increased deep tendon reflexes, muscle spasm, muscle cramps, paresthesias, and muscle twitching. X-ray findings of bone may include increased bone density.

Hypoparathyroidism results in the body pulling calcium from the bone and increased amounts of calcium are found in circulation. Hypercalcemia is, therefore, usually always present and the first clue to the disease. The disease more commonly affects middle-aged women. As a result of calcium depletion from the bones, weakening of the bone structure can occur, and fractures ensue. Other orthopedic signs and symptoms of this metabolic disorder are muscle weakness, muscle fatigability, pain, decreased bone density on x-ray, and decreased muscle tone. Treatment is similar to that of osteoporosis with correction of hypercalcemia.

Rickets

Rickets is a metabolic disorder caused by vitamin D deficiency. Rickets is most common in infants and in developing countries. In the United States, it can be observed in dark-skinned children, children with little sunlight exposure, vegetarian children that exclude dairy products, and sometimes breast-fed infants. Signs and symptoms of rickets may include those associated with the failure-to-thrive, bowing of long bones, forehead protrusion, palpable knots between the ribs, x-ray findings of increased epiphyseal space, and later signs of hypocalcemia may occur. Treatment is avoided at prevention and vitamin D supplementation.

Chvostek's sign and Trousseau's phenomenon

Chvostek's sign: this sign is used to assess the paresthesias often found in the individual with hypoparathyroidism and hypocalcemia. To perform this test, the examiner taps over the facial nerve of the patient (on the side of the cheekbone). A positive Chvostek's sign is elicited if the patient demonstrates muscle twitches around the eyes, nose and mouth with the tapping.

Trousseau's phenomenon: this test is used to assess tetany often found with hypoparathyroidism and hypocalcemia. Tightening and inflating a blood pressure cuff on the proximal forearm and leaving it in place for 3 minutes perform the test. The Trousseau's phenomenon results when this causes the wrist and MCP joints to flex and the fingers to abduct.

Oncology

Osteosarcoma

Osteosarcoma is a malignant tumor of the bone, most commonly seen in children. It primarily affects the long bones. Osteosarcoma can reoccur and metastasis to the lungs is common. Signs of osteosarcoma are children complaining of bone or extremity pain. The pain is often severe enough to awake them at night. There may be a palpable mass in the area of pain, and eventually it may cause altered use of the limb. Osteosarcoma is initially suspected on x-ray, then usually confirmed with biopsy. MRI, CT scan and bone scans may be performed to rule out metastasis. Management includes surgical removal and chemotherapy. Prognosis is good is the osteosarcoma has not spread. The patient can regain full use and function of the limb with rehabilitation. Regular follow up screening is necessary to detect osteosarcoma reoccurrence.

Soft-tissue sarcoma

Soft-tissue sarcomas are always malignant tumors that form from connective tissue, fat, muscle fibers and nerves. This tumor can affect any part of the body. The sarcoma can be localized or it may metastasize. A larger percentage of soft-tissue sarcomas are found in males and in the extremities. There are several types of soft-tissue sarcoma, but malignant fibrous histiocytoma is among the most common. A common initial complaint of these soft-tissue tumors is a visible or palpable growing mass. Definitive diagnosis is by biopsy, but a number of other imaging techniques may be used.

Metastatic bone disease

Metastatic bone disease is by far the most common bone cancer seen. It is usually seen later in life when primary cancers from the lungs, kidneys, breasts, and prostate spread. Bone metastasis is commonly seen in the axial skeleton and proximal long bones. The patient history is similar to many musculoskeletal conditions, but maintain a high-index of suspicion if there is a history of cancer. Anemia is present on blood work and imaging studies such as plain films, MRI and bone scan lend to the diagnosis. Treatment is usually surgical excision.

Multiple myeloma

Multiple myeloma is a malignant tumor that arises from bone marrow. There seems to be a genetic predisposition for this cancer. It affects both sexes equally and usually appears later in life, after 50. The patient complains of bone pain primarily, with secondary symptoms of anemia that are commonly found with the diagnosis of multiple myeloma. Other nonspecific lab findings are increased calcium, ESR, creatinine and BUN with decreased platelets. Bone marrow biopsy is the most sensitive diagnostic test. Treatment is primarily with chemotherapy, although bone marrow transplant may be considered for younger patients. Survival varies greatly on early diagnosis and patient health; however, the median survival for multiple myeloma is 2 years. Complications include: skeletal deformity from bone marrow destruction, immunosuppresion, fractures, and the development of amyloidosis.

Musculoskeletal tumor surgical interventions

Intralesional excision: this type of surgical procedure may also be termed curettage or intracpsular excision. This is commonly used if a total resection is

not an option, such as in metastatic bone disease. It is also commonly used for benign tumors.
Marginal excision: this may also be termed simple excision. This is usually saved for benign tumors. Surgical removal of the tumor right up to its borders is done, until borders tissue/cells are no longer reactive like those in the tumor. This leaves normal tissue in place.
Wide excision: this type of surgical procedures is more likely to be done with osteosarcomas. The tumor itself is removed in addition to a wide border of surrounding healthy tissue.
Radical resection: this surgical procedure removes the tumor and the entire structure that contains the tumor (bone or muscle). This is commonly done in advanced stage osteosarcomas.

Tumor staging methods

Tumor staging is necessary to classify the degree of malignancy. It helps guide medical management and determine prognosis. The staging involves assessing tumor involve using three main components, and then further placing a score on these. The first component is determining the grade (G) of the tumor. The grade is classified as high or low, high being without clearly defined borders and high risk of metastasis and low describing a well-demarcated tumor with low risk of spread. The second component of classification is the tumor site (T). Again the site description is further labeled with a 1 or 2. A T1 labeling indicates a well-contained tumor. The label T2 suggests the tumor travels beyond the anatomical compartment. Finally, staging identifies metastasis (M), using M0 to show no metastasis, M1 indicates local spread, and sometimes M3 is used to identify distant metastases.

Practice Test

Practice Questions

1. Which of the following conditions is a CONTRAINDICATION for use of the supine sling?
   a. Osteoporosis with degenerative disk disease
   b. Rheumatoid arthritis
   c. Severe respiratory compromise
   d. Stroke with hemiplegia

2. Which of the following is the most common treatment for carpal tunnel syndrome?
   a. Corticosteroid injections
   b. Stretching exercises
   c. Splinting
   d. Surgical repair

3. Which of the following is the correct position for the patient during application of a figure-8 clavicle strap for a right clavicular fracture?
   a. Sitting in upright attention position
   b. Leaning forward
   c. Supine
   d. Left-lying

4. A 30-year-old patient in good physical condition with a non-weight-bearing cast is preparing for discharge. Which method of ambulation is usually indicated?
   a. Ambulation with 4-wheeled Roll-A-Bout® walker
   b. Ambulation with pickup or 2-wheeled walker
   c. Crutch walking, 3-point gait
   d. Crutch walking, 4-point gait

5. A pediatric fracture of a long bone classified as Salter-Harris Type V results in:
   a. No impairment in growth
   b. Excess bone growth
   c. Growth disturbance
   d. Growth arrest

6. Which of the following is a CONTRAINDICATION to bisphosphonate therapy?
   a. Hypercalcemia
   b. Hypocalcemia
   c. Hyperphosphatemia
   d. Hypophosphatemia

7. A patient with a stable fractured sacrum is primarily at increased risk for which of the following?
   a. Avascular necrosis
   b. Fat embolism
   c. Paralytic ileus
   d. Deep vein thrombosis

8. A 17-year-old adolescent injures his left knee during a football game. He is in severe pain and the knee has obvious deformity, but the posterior tibial and dorsal pulses are palpable. Which, if any, is the appropriate initial splinting procedure?
   a. Leg splinted straight with knee in proper position
   b. Knee splinted in position found
   c. Knee splinted against opposite knee for stability
   d. Knee cushioned but not splinted

9. Which of the following is CONTRAINDICATED for the operative leg following hip replacement surgery?
   a. Adduction
   b. Abduction
   c. Hip flexion $\leq 90°$
   d. External rotation

10. Following total knee replacement, a 50-year-old male's leg is placed in a continuous passive motion (CPM) device with initial settings at 10 degrees extension and 50 degrees flexion. What is the usual extension/flexion goal for discharge?
   a. 10 degrees extension, 70 degrees flexion
   b. 0 degrees extension, 90 degrees flexion
   c. 5 degrees extension, 80 degrees flexion
   d. 10 degrees extension and 90 degrees flexion

11. A patient with osteoporosis suffered two fractured ribs as a result of a fall. Which is the most appropriate measure to promote comfort during deep breathing and coughing exercises?
   a. Chest strapping with immobilization
   b. Holding a pillow against the chest
   c. Wrapping arms about the chest to splint
   d. Lying flat on the bed

12. A 55-year-old patient has a swollen knee with 3+ joint effusion, tenderness, decreased ROM, and increased skin temperature on palpation. Which of the following tests is most accurate in differentiating septic arthritis from inflammatory synovitis?
   a. Radiograph
   b. White blood count with differential
   c. Erythrocyte sedimentation rate
   d. Aspiration of joint

13. A cross-country runner has experienced repeated anterior shin splints. Which of the following interventions is indicated to prevent further episodes?
  a. Arch supports, heel lifts, and stretching the calf muscles
  b. Enforced period of rest and slow return to activity
  c. Supportive splint on ankle and lower leg
  d. Orthotic arch supports and reducing stride

14. A 45-year-old male, who had been moving heavy boxes, developed poorly-localized moderate dull aching pain in the lower back, radiating into the right buttock. Which of the following initial treatments is most appropriate?
  a. Opioid and activity restriction for 5 days
  b. NSAID and resumption of moderate activity
  c. NSAID and physical therapy
  d. Muscle relaxant and bed rest for at least 5 days

15. An 18-year-old woman of small stature suffered severe lacerations and open fractures of the tibia and fibula as the result of a severe mauling by an unidentified Rottweiler dog that was not captured. Which of the following is NOT required?
  a. Rabies post-exposure prophylaxis (PEP)
  b. Tetanus toxoid/tetanus immune globulin as indicated
  c. Antibiotic prophylaxis
  d. Antiinflammatory drugs (NSAIDs)

16. A patient with acute olecranon bursitis is treated with RICE therapy and NSAID for discomfort. What should the patient be advised about use of the elbow?
  a. Immobilize the joint for about one week and then avoid all aggravating activities for 1 to 2 weeks
  b. Use the elbow moderately for 1 week and then increase use to tolerance
  c. Immobilize the elbow until all symptoms subside
  d. Do ROM exercises at least 4 times daily and continue with moderate use

17. A 65-year-old woman with osteoporosis needs to increase calcium in the diet. Which of the following foods has the highest calcium content?
  a. 1 cup fat-free milk
  b. 1 cup cottage cheese
  c. 1 tablespoon blackstrap molasses
  d. 1 cup cooked kale

18. A 25-year-old woman fell on an outstretched arm, resulting in a posterior dislocation of the elbow. After reduction, the elbow was placed through range of motion without problem, x-rayed, and then immobilized with a splint in 90° flexion. One-half hour later, examination shows mild vascular compromise in the hand. Which initial action is most appropriate?
  a. Prepare patient for surgical intervention
  b. Remove splint
  c. Take repeat radiograph
  d. Loosen splint and/or lessen flexion

19. A 66-year-old diabetic male develops osteomyelitis with erythema, edema, pain and purulent discharge in the tibia at the site of a previous traumatic injury. Which of the following is generally CONTRAINDICATED during initial treatment?

a. IV antibiotics
b. Gentle ROM exercises of knee and ankle
c. Immobilization device (splint)
d. Full weight bearing

20. Which of the following fractures places the patient most at risk of life-threatening hemorrhage?

a. Knee
b. Tibia
c. Pelvis
d. Fibula

21. A 20-year-old male soccer player developed peroneus brevis tendinitis and is treated initially with RICE and non-weight bearing. Which of the following is CONTRAINDICATED?

a. Using heel lifts and lateral sole wedge
b. Going barefoot or wearing low-heeled shoes
c. Strengthening exercises
d. NSAIDs

22. Which of the following is CONTRAINDICATED as initial treatment for epicondylitis (tennis elbow)?

a RICE
b. NSAID
c. Immobilization
d. Corticosteroid injection

23. Parents report that their 8-month-old child fell when trying to stand. Radiographs show the infant has a spiral fracture of the humerus. Which of the following does this suggest?

a. Neglect
b. Abuse
c. Lack of adequate nutrition
d. Bone disorder

24. A 58-year-old patient with Lambert-Eaton myasthenic syndrome (LEMS) has the highest risk for which of the following?

a. Respiratory failure
b. Cancer
c. Blindness
d. Weight gain

25. A 55-year-old male had palmar and digital fasciectomies to correct the flexion deformity associated with Dupuytren's contracture. Which of the following topics for home care instruction is most critical?
   a. Finger exercises
   b. Neurovascular assessment
   c. Medication use
   d. Infection control

26. Which of the following is NOT necessary for a patient with moderate erosive rheumatoid arthritis?
   a. Nutrition therapy
   b. Occupational therapy
   c. Reconstructive surgery
   d. Physical therapy

27. A 62-year-old male with Paget's disease has a thickened skull with possible cranial nerve compression. For which of the following should the patient be initially assessed?
   a. Hearing loss
   b. Difficulty swallowing
   c. Vision impairment
   d. Cognitive impairment

28. A 13-year-old girl with scoliosis of 38 degrees is required to wear a brace for 23 hours daily but has repeatedly removed the brace before leaving for school. Which of the following is the best initial strategy?
   a. Explain the importance of wearing the brace
   b. Develop a list of punishments for not wearing the brace
   c. Tell the parents to check the brace each morning before the child leaves
   d. Show the girl how to dress to minimize the appearance of the brace

29. A 10-year-old boy develops sharp knee pain while playing basketball. Pain worsens when walking up and down stairs. X-rays show damage to the growth plate of the tibial tuberosity, consistent with Osgood-Schlatter syndrome. Which of the following is the primary treatment?
   a. Stopping physical activities for 7 days and then gradually resuming
   b. Applying cast to immobilize the knee
   c. Cortisone injection into the knee joint
   d. Oral anti-inflammatory medications

30. A 60-year-old woman with osteoporosis asks for information about reducing the risk of fractures. She has a diet high in calcium and vitamin D and takes supplements as prescribed. She smokes 1 pack of cigarettes, drinks 1 glass of wine, and walks 2 miles daily outdoors. Which of the following interventions is most essential to reducing risk?
   a. Increasing weight-bearing exercise
   b. Stopping use of alcohol
   c. Dietary instruction
   d. Smoking cessation

31. A 55-year-old male with polymyalgia rheumatica and giant cell arteritis states that he plans to stop taking corticosteroids because of weight gain. Which of the following should the nurse stress as the most important reason to continue treatment?
a. To reduce joint swelling
b. To prevent blindness
c. To increase strength
d. To reduce pain and stiffness

32. Which initial medication is preferred for a first acute attack of gout with inflammation of the right great toe and elevated uric acid level?
a. Colchicine
b. Probenecid
c. NSAID
d. Allopurinol

33. A patient with a long-leg cast complains of pain in the lateral knee area. On examination, the cast is discolored below the knee and a slight odor is present. However, the pulse and circulation in the foot are good. Which of the following complications is most consistent with these signs/symptoms?
a. Compartment syndrome
b. Pressure ulcer
c. Fat embolism
d. Disuse syndrome

34. A 14-year-old boy was diagnosed with osteosarcoma of the distal femur. Because of extensive neurovascular spread, he was not a candidate for a limb-sparing procedure but had an AK amputation and chemotherapy (preoperative and postoperative). Although receiving counseling, he has become increasingly angry and uncooperative, shouting that he wished he had died and is a freak. Which of the following is the best strategy?
a. Ignore his outbursts
b. Use positive reinforcement to reward him for good behavior
c. Engage him in self-care and decision-making
d. Change to a different counselor

35. Which of the following interventions may reduce pain associated with Morton's neuroma?
a. Shoe with soft padded innersoles
b. Shoe with heel lift
c. Rigid ankle-foot orthosis
d. Shoe with innersole and metatarsal pad

36. The nurse is providing discharge education for parents of a 2-month-old infant diagnosed with osteogenesis imperfecta, Type IV, after an arm fracture. Which is the best method to transport the child from hospital to home?
a. Holding the infant on a foam pad of pillow
b. Sitting in a standard car seat
c. Reclining in a padded car seat
d. Lying flat in a secured and padded bassinet

37. A 28-year-old female long-distance runner developed a tibial stress fracture and has been on restricted activity for 8 weeks. Which of the following topics for patient education is most important to help her prevent further injury?
a. Nutrition therapy
b. Training procedures
c. Muscle strengthening
d. Body mechanics

38. Which of the following is NOT a risk factor for osteoporosis?
a. History of childhood wrist fracture
b. Cushing's syndrome
c. Small skeletal frame
d. History of post-menopausal vertebral fracture

39. Which of the following interventions is NOT recommended for patients with osteoarthritis to help manage pain and improve mobility?
a. Acupressure/acupuncture
b. Application of cold packs to joints
c. Guided imagery and progressive muscle relaxation
d. Tai Chi class

40. Which of the following is CONTRAINDICATED in the postoperative period of a lumbar laminectomy?
a. Using the logrolling technique for turning
b. Sitting for 30 minutes
c. Lying flat in bed with knees slightly elevated
d. Having the patient assist in turning by holding onto the side rail

41. Which of the following is most commonly associated with degenerative disk disease?
a. Kyphosis
b. Lordosis
c. Scoliosis
d. Gibbus deformity

42. Which of the following is an example of a first exercise following surgical repair of a rotator cuff tear?
a. Slowly raising the extended arm to 90 degrees
b. Lifting a bar upward with arm extended to the side
c. Bending over and allowing the arm to dangle and swing in circles
d. Raising and lowering 2-pound weights with arm extended

43. A 34-year-old male ruptured his Achilles tendon while playing football. Which of the following is the primary advantage of surgical repair over conservative medical treatment with casting?
a. Lower rate of rerupture
b. Lower rate of infection
c. Less pain
d. Faster recovery period

44. Which of the following should patients receiving methotrexate for treatment of rheumatoid arthritis restrict?

a. Smoking
b. Alcohol
c. Sodium
d. Fluid intake

45. A 22-year-old female returning from war with a traumatic BK amputation of her left arm has phantom pain that has been unrelieved by opioids, antidepressants, anticonvulsants, and nerve stimulation. Which of the following interventions is the most appropriate to try next?

a. Mirror box
b. Acupuncture
c. Brain stimulation
d. Stump revision

46. A 25-year-old patient with multiple fractures from an auto accident develops hypoxia, dyspnea, precordial chest pain, tachycardia, and thick milky sputum. Auscultation of the lungs shows crackles and wheezes. The patient complains of headache and has a fever of 40°C. Which of the following interventions should be done first?

a. High-flow oxygen
b. Corticosteroids (IV)
c. Vasopressors
d. Morphine

47. A 70-year-old woman fell on an open and dorsiflexed hand, resulting in a fracture of the distal radius. Two days after closed reduction and application of a short-arm cast, the patient took a shower and got the proximal part of the cast damp. Which initial intervention is indicated?

a. Removal and reapplication of the cast
b. Drying the cast with hair dryer on cool setting
c. Allowing the cast to air dry only
d. Replacing the cast with a splint

48. Which of the following is NOT one of the 3 components of the female athlete triad?

a. Eating disorder
b. Osteoporosis
c. Overuse syndrome
d. Amenorrhea

49. Which position is usually best to relieve acute low back pain?

a. Side-lying curled position with knees and hips flexed and pillow separating knees
b. Sitting upright in a soft chair
c. Standing at a walker with weight supported by extending arms
d. Lying prone

50. Concurrent administration of which of the following increases gastrointestinal toxicity and bleeding related to long-term NSAID therapy?

a. Proton pump inhibitor
b. Antacid
c. Acetaminophen
d. Steroid

Answers and Explanations

1. C: The supine sling is contraindicated for patients with severe respiratory compromise because it precludes elevation of the head and may increase respiratory distress. The supine sling can be used with almost any other patient, especially those who must remain flat or cannot tolerate more upright positions. The supine sling is used for lateral transfers, bathing, repositioning, changing linen, rescuing after a fall, and transferring of a deceased patient. Supine slings may be padded or unpadded and may be made of mesh to facilitate bathing.

2. C: The most common treatment for carpal tunnel syndrome is splinting to maintain the wrist in a neutral position and prevent further compression of the nerve. Carpel tunnel syndrome occurs when the median nerve is compressed within the carpel tunnel, formed from ligaments, tendons, and bones, between the forearm and the hand. Initial symptoms include numbness, tingling, or burning in the hand, especially the palm, thumb, and index and middle fingers, with eventual weakening and inability to grip. Compression increases when the wrist is flexed, so the symptoms may worsen during sleep. Corticosteroid injections are usually now avoided because they may result in nerve damage or scarring. Gentle stretching may reduce pain.

3. A: The patient should sit upright in attention position for application of the figure-8 clavicle strap, as this keeps bones in proper alignment; however, the patient may require pain medication prior to assuming this position and may need to assume the position slowly. Prior to application of the strap, the arm and hand on the fracture side should be assessed for neurological or vascular impairment, noting color, temperature, sensation, numbness or tingling, motor function, and strength of pulses.

4. C: A patient in good physical condition with a non-weight-bearing cast is usually instructed in crutch walking with a 3-point gait. The 4-point gait is used with a partial-weight-bearing cast. Elderly patients and patients with poor balance or an inability to use crutches may use walkers. Two-wheeled or pickup walkers are easy to control, but ambulation is slower, as the person must step toward the walker, advance the walker, and then step again. The Roll-A-Bout walker may be used for those who are unable to manage crutches, but it requires weight bearing on the knee.

5. D: Salter-Harris Type V pediatric fractures are characterized by crushing trauma to the epiphyseal plate with growth arrest. Other classifications are the following:

- Fracture goes through the growth plate, but prognosis is good.
- Fracture goes through the growth plate and into the metaphysis, but prognosis is good.
- Fracture goes through the growth plate and into the epiphysis, and growth disturbance may occur.
- Fracture goes through the growth plate, epiphysis, and metaphysis, and growth disturbance may occur.

6. B: Hypocalcemia is a contraindication because bisphosphonates induce hypocalcemia and will worsen the condition. More than 99% of calcium (Ca) is in the skeletal system with 1% in serum, but it is important for transmitting nerve impulses and regulating contraction and relaxation of the muscles, including the myocardium. Calcium levels should be monitored periodically during bisphosphonate therapy, and any indication of hypocalcemia, such as tetany, tingling, seizures, altered mental status, and ventricular tachycardia should be treated with calcium and vitamin D supplementation.
Normal values: 8.2 to 10.2 mg/dL
Hypocalcemia: <8.2. Critical value: <7 mg/dL
Hypercalcemia: >10.2 mg/dL. Critical value: >12 mg/dL

7. C: A fractured sacrum is associated with increased risk of paralytic ileus, so the patient's bowel sounds should be monitored frequently. A stable pelvic structure (including a fractured sacrum) usually heals fairly rapidly because the blood supply is good; however, pelvic fractures increase risk of fat embolism and DVT from inactivity. Avascular necrosis may occur with any bone if the blood supply is disrupted, but it is most common in the shoulder, hip (femoral head), and knee.

8. B: If there is considerable deformity but a posterior tibial pulse/dorsal pedal is still evident, then no attempt should be made to straighten the leg; it should be splinted in the position found to prevent further injury. Both dislocations and fractures have similar symptoms—pain, edema, deformity—but the pain with dislocation is often acute and severe, while pain related to knee fracture may be more obvious on palpation. Patellar dislocations are a less severe injury than knee dislocation and may result from twisting injuries or blunt trauma, and there is less pronounced deformity than with a knee dislocation.

9. A: Adduction is contraindicated after hip replacement surgery as it may result in dislocation of the prosthesis. The patient should be advised to maintain abduction by keeping the knees separated when sitting and placing a pillow between the knees when in bed. Flexion should not exceed 90°, so the patient must avoid bending to reach for items, to dress, or to sit on a toilet (which should be elevated). Internal rotation of the hip may also result in dislocation.

10. B: The extension/flexion goal is 0 degrees extension (full) and 90 degrees flexion. The purpose of the CPM device is to promote circulation, decrease incidence of complications (such as thromboembolia), and increase ROM. The CPM device is applied after surgery and should be used as much as possible in the initial postoperative period, although the patient is encouraged to begin ambulation, with the knee immobilized and restricted weight-bearing, within a day of surgery. The leg should be elevated when the patient is sitting.

11. B: The best method for the patient to use to splint the chest for DB&C exercises is to hold a pillow against the chest, as this provides some support, but not immobilization. Strapping the chest is no longer used with fractured ribs, because restriction increases risk of atelectasis and pneumonia. A second person may use hands to support the chest when the patient coughs, but if the patient wraps the arms about the chest, this may restrict ventilation. Lying flat in bed is not effective.

12. D: The most accurate test for differentiating septic arthritis from inflammatory synovitis is joint aspiration with gross and microscopic analysis of aspirant. With septic arthritis, the fluid is turbid to frankly purulent. Non-inflammatory effusions result in clear fluid, and inflammatory effusions in turbid fluid. WBC may increase with a left shift with septic arthritis, but septic arthritis can occur without WBC elevation. The ESR increases with both inflammatory and septic arthritis. Radiographs show changes in the bony structures but cannot differentiate inflammatory synovitis from septic arthritis.

13. D: The athlete may need orthotic arch supports to provide better support to the foot and must reduce stride to decrease the pull on the muscle. Runners with high arches have decreased shock absorption, so force is transmitted to the lateral aspect of the foot, radiating to the leg and knee and causing anterior shin splints (inflammation of the tibialis anterior muscle and connecting tendons). This induces pain in the shin area when running. Runners with low arches are prone to posterior shin splints, as excess force is transmitted to the medial aspects of the leg. Stretching the calf muscles, firm arch supports, and heel lifts may alleviate symptoms.

14. B: Dull, aching pain in the lower back radiating to the buttocks or thigh (but not below the knee) usually indicates musculoskeletal pain and is treated with NSAIDs and resumption of moderate activity. If pain is severe, initial bed rest of 1 or 2 days may be indicated, but early activity and pain control are usually as effective as physical therapy. Muscle relaxants are sometimes prescribed, although their effectiveness is not supported by research. Heat or cold therapy may provide some pain relief. Pain resulting from nerve compression is usually severe, localized, and shooting, with pain or numbness consistent with dermatomal distribution. Pain may be more severe in the leg than in the back.

15. D: Antiinflammatory drugs may be used to reduce discomfort, but they are not required after a dog bite with resultant soft tissue and skeletal injury. Rabies PEP must be given, because the dog was not captured and no information is available regarding rabies status. Tetanus immune globulin or a tetanus booster may be indicated if the most recent injection was >5 years earlier. Animal bites pose increased risk of infection and osteomyelitis, so antibiotic prophylaxis is routinely provided.

16. A: The elbow should be immobilized for about a week and then protected from activities that aggravate the elbow for at least one to two weeks. Using the elbow during the initial period may worsen the bursitis. The patient should be cautioned to increase activities slowly and avoid repetitive actions, overuse, resting weight on the elbows, and clenching the fists or holding items with a tight grip. Elbow pads may help avoid further injury when the patient resumes activities.

17. A: Milk products are high in calcium. One cup of fat-free milk contains about 300 mg of calcium, while cottage cheese has about 150 mg. One tablespoon of blackstrap molasses contains 172 mg, while 1 cup of cooked kale contains 179 mg. Dairy products, soy products, calcium-fortified cereals and juices, canned fish (salmon, sardines), and green leafy vegetables are good sources of calcium. In order to utilize calcium, vitamin D levels must also be adequate, and milk products are often fortified with vitamin D.

18. D: Mild vascular compromise in the hand can usually be relieved by loosening the splint or slightly lessening flexion to improve circulation. Inability to place the elbow through

ROM may indicate a medial epicondyle fracture that requires surgical intervention; however, ROM was successful after reduction. Completely removing the splint is not indicated as maintaining the bones in proper alignment after a dislocation is necessary to prevent redislocation and to allow healing. A second radiograph is not warranted at this time.

19. D: Full weight bearing is contraindicated with osteomyelitis because the infection weakens the bone, sometimes resulting in pathologic fracture. An immobilization device (such as a splint) is applied to decrease pain and protect the bone. IV antibiotics are started as soon as culture is sent to the laboratory in order to reduce infection before thrombosis occurs. Most infections result from Staphylococcus aureus, but if culture shows other organisms, the initial antibiotic may be changed after culture and sensitivity testing. The joints above/below the infected area should be put through gentle ROM.

20. C: While substantial blood loss may occur with fractures, those involving the pelvis or bilateral femurs put the patient most at risk for life-threatening hemorrhage. With pelvis or long-bone fractures, two large-bore IV lines should be in place for fluid replacement. Estimated blood loss amounts with fractures are as follows:

- Elbow, tibial, ankle: 0.5 to 1.5 L
- Femur: 1 to 2 L
- Forearm: 0.5 to 1 L
- Hip: 1.5 to 2.5 L
- Pelvis: 1.5 to 4.5 L
- Tibia: 0.5 to 1.5

21. B: A patient recovering from peroneus brevis tendinitis should avoid going barefoot or wearing low-heeled shoes, as this increases the load on the tendon. The peroneus brevis tendon stabilizes the foot and usually prevents lateral sprain, but if sprain occurs, the tendon can be injured with resultant tendinitis, tear, or rupture. Heel lifts relieve load, and a lateral sole wedge prevents the foot from rolling laterally. Physical therapy may include strengthening, proprioception, and flexibility exercises. Pain is controlled with NSAIDs.

22. D: Corticosteroid injection is contraindicated as an initial treatment, because corticosteroids may cause a degenerative effect in the tendon; however, if initial treatments, such as RICE therapy and NSAID, are not effective and pain remains severe, corticosteroid injection may be used. Some patients are treated with immobilization with a splint or cast, depending on severity of tendinitis and degree of pain on movement. Stretching exercises usually begin after pain subsides. Patients may be advised to use a counterforce strap when they begin playing tennis again.

23. B: A spiral fracture of a long bone, especially in a child <9 months, is often an indication of child abuse in which someone has twisted the child's arm. Children fall many times when learning to walk, but this rarely results in fractures, so allowing a child to fall when trying to stand is not a sign of neglect. While poor nutrition and some bone disorders can result in weak bones, a spiral fracture is not common. The child should be carefully examined for evidence of previous injuries.

24. C: LEMS is commonly paraneoplastic with over 80% of patients developing cancer, primarily small-cell lung cancer, breast cancer, GI cancers, and ovarian cancer. Respiratory depression is rarely severe with LEMS, and vision impairment relates to diplopia and ptosis. Weight loss is common. Patients typically experience weakness in proximal muscles. While symptoms are similar to myasthenia gravis (MG), electromyography can differentiate the two. With LEMS, muscle power increases with prolonged contraction, whereas it decreases with MG.

25. B: Teaching the patient to monitor neurovascular status is of critical importance to prevent complications. Assessment should include skin temperature, capillary refill, sensation, motor function, and response to pain medication, as unrelieved pain may indicate neurovascular compromise. Use of medication to control pain should also be reviewed, as well as control of edema by elevating the hand. This may relieve pain and reduce the incidence of neurovascular complications. Monitoring for signs of infection and using methods to prevent infection are also important.

26. C: Reconstructive surgery is reserved for persistent erosive RA, but in the early stages, other therapies are indicated. Occupational therapy: Joint protection, overuse avoidance, and activity pacing are indicated to help the patient remain independent in activities of daily living. Physical therapy: ROM and muscle strengthening help to slow progress of the disease and to maintain strength and mobility. Nutrition therapy: Because anemia and anorexia are common, the patient needs therapy to help identify eating habits and to ensure that the diet is adequate. If the patient is on corticosteroids, which increase appetite, calorie restriction may be appropriate.

27. A: Paget's disease, a disorder associated with rapid bone turnover in localized areas (skull, femur, pelvic bones, tibia, vertebrae), may cause thickening of the skull and compression of the facial nerves. Skull involvement is often associated with loss of hearing, so patients should be assessed for hearing loss and fitted with hearing aids and provided education in alternative communication methods, such as speech reading and body language, if indicated. Fractures and degenerative arthritis are also common, so patients should have diets high in calcium and vitamin D.

28. D: The best approach to ensuring compliance with wearing of the brace for scoliosis is to validate the girl's feelings and discuss the types of clothes to wear to minimize the appearance of the brace. A girl in early adolescence is often more concerned about immediate social issues than long-term health issues, such as the reasons for wearing the brace. Punishment or parental monitoring is likely to increase resentment and may cause the child to rebel further.

29. A: The primary treatment for Osgood-Schlatter syndrome is to instruct the child to stop all physical activities, such as running and jumping, for at least a week and then to gradually resume activities over the next month or so to prevent recurrence of symptoms. Immobilizing the knee does not aid in healing, but a temporary splint may provide some relief of pain. While NSAIDs may be used to relieve discomfort, a cortisone injection into the knee is not indicated. Symptoms may recur in some children.

30. D: Smoking cessation is most important to reduce the risk of fractures, because smoking reduces osteogenesis. While alcohol has a similar effect, moderate drinking (1 glass of wine daily) is acceptable. A diet high in calcium and vitamin D and supplements are standard preventive treatments, as is outdoor exposure to sunlight to increase absorption of vitamin D. Weight-bearing exercises are essential, and 30 minutes daily is recommended. Most people walk about 20 minutes/mile, so the patient's daily walk exceeds this goal and also provides exposure to sunlight.

31. B: Strict adherence to corticosteroid protocol is essential with giant cell arteritis (associated with polymyalgia rheumatica) to prevent complications, such as a sudden, permanent loss of vision. Moderate doses of corticosteroid are used for polymyalgia rheumatica alone. Corticosteroids reduce joint swelling (usually mild) and the pain and stiffness associated with polymyalgia rheumatica. Proximal muscle pain is most acute, especially in the neck, shoulder, and pelvis, and stiffness is most noticeable in the early morning and after periods of inactivity.

32. C: Gout (metabolic arthritis) is usually treated first with NSAIDs. If patients are unable to tolerate NSAIDs, then colchicine may be prescribed. Probenecid (to prevent tophi formation) and allopurinol (to prevent formation of uric acid) may be used for chronic episodes. Other treatments include restriction of high purine food (organ meats), and alcohol and weight reduction. Gout is associated with a defect of purine metabolism that results in hyperuricemia, with oversecretion of uric acid, decreased excretion of uric acid, or a combination. The increased uric acid levels (>7 mg/dL) can cause monosodium urate crystal deposits in the joints, resulting in severe articular and periarticular inflammation.

33. B: These signs/symptoms are consistent with a pressure ulcer. A window may be cut into the cast, or the cast may be bi-valved so the area can be examined and treated. Compartment syndrome is characterized by impaired circulation and is treated by bi-valving the cast and elevating the limb. If symptoms persist, a fasciotomy is needed. Fat embolism results in systemic effects, such as hypoxia, tachypnea, fever, and tachycardia and is an emergent condition. Disuse syndrome results in atrophy and weakness of muscles and is prevented by muscle-setting exercises (such as quadriceps and gluteal setting).

34. C: Engaging the adolescent in self-care and decision-making is the best strategy to deal with his anger, a normal stage in the grieving process. He is trying to adjust to changes in his body image at a critical time in his development and may feel he has no control over his life or his body. Stating, "I can see that you're angry" and validating his feelings is better than ignoring outbursts. While positive reinforcement may have a place in rehabilitation, his behavior is neither good nor bad but a sign of emotional distress. Because this behavior is normal, a change in counselors is probably not necessary.

35. D: Wearing a shoe with an innersole and a metatarsal pad to spread the metatarsal heads may relieve pressure on the nerves. With Morton's neuroma, impingement of the plantar nerve causes the nerve to become inflamed and enlarged. Flat feet or wearing of high heels may compress the nerve between the bones (usually the third and fourth metatarsals), resulting in inflammation with pain and numbness. Neuromas or benign

tumors of the plantar digital nerves in the webbed areas between the toes may also cause pressure on the nerve. Athletes (such as golfers) who spin on the ball of the foot are prone to this disorder.

36. C: Laws require that infants be secured in a car seat, so holding the infant and transporting in a bassinet are precluded. The best method is to use a car seat that reclines and to pad it with egg-crate foam so the child is on a soft and cushioned surface. The parents should also be cautioned to place padding between the infant's trunk and the securing straps, as they may cause fractures if fastened tightly against the child's trunk.

37. B: Training procedures should be reviewed in detail, as most stress fractures result from errors in training, such as increasing training too quickly and wearing improperly-fitted or inadequately-supportive shoes. Shoes should be replaced frequently, at least every 500 km, and should be well cushioned. Athletes with flat feet may require orthoses for arch support. The patient should start activity by walking and slowly progress to jogging and running. A nutritious diet high in calcium, muscle-strengthening exercises, and proper body mechanics may also improve conditioning.

38. A: A childhood wrist fracture is not a risk factor for osteoporosis; however, a post-menopausal vertebral fracture poses considerable risk of further fractures. Women who have a small frame and low weight tend to have lower bone density and increased risk. A number of diseases increase risk of osteoporosis: diabetes mellitus, hyperparathyroidism, Cushing's syndrome, and Addison's disease. Medications, such as corticosteroids, also increase risk. Other risk factors include female gender, inadequate exercise, excessive drinking, smoking, reduced estrogen level, inadequate calcium and/or vitamin D, advanced age, and race (21% incidence in Caucasians and 18% in Hispanics).

39. B: Cold may reduce pain in inflammatory joint disorders if joints are swollen and erythematous, but osteoarthritis is usually relieved by heat application. The nurse should instruct all patients with osteoarthritis in guided imagery and progressive muscle relaxation, as studies show this reduces pain and increases mobility. Acupressure or acupuncture may benefit some patients by reducing pain. Tai Chi, which involves slow movement and stretching, can also help maintain flexibility and reduce pain.

40. D: Any activity that strains the lower back may cause herniation after surgery, so the patient should not hold onto the side rails to assist in turning and should avoid bending from the waist, lifting (> 5 lb.), and twisting movements for at least the first 2 weeks. When lying in bed (flat or with a small pillow), slightly elevating the knees may reduce pressure on the lower back and increase comfort. Patients should avoid complete bed rest but should also avoid prolonged sitting of ≥45 minutes.

41. A: Kyphosis (convex curvature), also called "dowager's hump," is most-commonly associated with degenerative disk disease and occurs in post-menopausal women. Scoliosis (lateral S-shaped curvature) may be congenital, neuromuscular, or idiopathic and is usually diagnosed during adolescence. Lordosis (concave curvature) often increases during

adolescence or early adulthood. Gibbus deformity is a form of kyphosis associated with skeletal tuberculosis.

42. C: Because only passive motion is permitted in the initial healing stage after surgery to repair a rotator cuff tear, bending over and allowing the arm to dangle and swing in circles helps to gently stretch the muscles and maintain flexibility. Most often, simple ROM exercises of the hand and wrist begin within 2 to 3 days of surgery, and dangling and wall-walking exercises begin at 7 to 10 days. Active motions, such as lifting the arm unaided or lifting other items, such as weights, must be avoided, as stress on the muscles may cause reinjury.

43. A: The primary advantage of surgical repair of a rupture of the Achilles tendon over conservative medical treatment is a lower rate of rerupture, which occurs in about 4% after surgery but ≥8% with conservative treatment. Percutaneous procedures are now available, but complication rates are higher than with open surgery. Infection is more common with surgery, and pain varies but may be comparable. Both procedures require extended recovery times, as surgery is followed by casting to prevent damage to the healing tendon.

44. B: Alcohol combined with methotrexate may increase hepatotoxic effects of the drug, so alcohol should be completely restricted or use strictly curtailed. Liver function tests should be done every 4 to 8 weeks during methotrexate therapy. Smoking should always be restricted for general health purposes. Fluid intake should be encouraged, and methotrexate does not require restriction of sodium; however, patients taking corticosteroids (which promote sodium retention) may benefit from restricting sodium intake to reduce fluid retention.

45. A: Since treatments should begin with the least invasive, the mirror box should be tried next to relieve phantom pain. The patient inserts her intact arm into one side of the box and her stump into the other side of the box. The box is separated by a center mirror. The patient then moves the intact arm and hand and observes the image reflected in the mirror, imagining that the image is her amputated limb. This "tricks" the brain into thinking the arm is intact and relieves pain in a significant number of people.

46. A: These symptoms are consistent with fat embolism syndrome (FES), which may cause rapid acute pulmonary edema and acute respiratory distress syndrome (ARDS), so the patient should be immediately provided with high-flow oxygen. Controlled-volume ventilation with positive-end expiratory pressure (PEEP) may be indicated to prevent/treat pulmonary edema. Corticosteroids may reduce inflammation of the lungs and reduce cerebral edema. Vasopressors prevent hypotension and interstitial pulmonary edema. Morphine with a benzodiazepine may be indicated for patients who require artificial ventilation.

47. B: Drying a cast can be difficult, but the best approach is to use a hair dryer on a cool setting. If the cast is extensively damaged or remains wet on the inside, it may need to be changed to prevent skin irritation or lack of adequate support. A splint is sometimes applied immediately after injury when there is swelling, but it is usually replaced with a cast to ensure that bones stay in correct alignment.

48. C: Overuse syndrome, although it may occur, is not a component of the female athlete triad, which comprises the following:
Eating disorder: This may include anorexia and/or bulimia, dietary restrictions, or use of diuretics and/or laxatives to control weight.
Amenorrhea (>3 months): Estrogen levels fall because of the effect excess exercise and weight fluctuations have on the hypothalamus and gonadotropic hormones.
Osteoporosis: Bone resorption increases because of the depressed levels of estrogen, resulting in decreased bone density and increased risk of fractures.

49. A: One of the best positions to relieve acute back pain is a side-lying curled position with knees and hips flexed and a pillow separating the knees, although patients should be encouraged to change position and alternate periods of sitting, standing, and lying. Positions that increase lordosis, such as the prone position, may increase pain for many people. Sitting should be done in a firm chair with arm support and a pillow at the back to facilitate standing. Some people find that lying on a firm surface with the head elevated to 30° and knees slightly elevated also reduces discomfort.

50. D: Steroids given concurrently with NSAIDs increase risk of GI toxicity and bleeding, so this is a particular problem for those with rheumatoid arthritis. NSAIDs should be administered with food. Concurrent administration of a proton pump inhibitor (such as omeprazole) or an antacid may reduce risk, although antacids may mask symptoms to some degree. Acetaminophen does not usually cause GI upset or bleeding, and the combination of an NSAID and acetaminophen may be more effective for pain control than the NSAID alone.

Secret Key #1 - Time is Your Greatest Enemy

Pace Yourself

Wear a watch. At the beginning of the test, check the time (or start a chronometer on your watch to count the minutes), and check the time after every few questions to make sure you are "on schedule."

If you are forced to speed up, do it efficiently. Usually one or more answer choices can be eliminated without too much difficulty. Above all, don't panic. Don't speed up and just begin guessing at random choices. By pacing yourself, and continually monitoring your progress against your watch, you will always know exactly how far ahead or behind you are with your available time. If you find that you are one minute behind on the test, don't skip one question without spending any time on it, just to catch back up. Take 15 fewer seconds on the next four questions, and after four questions you'll have caught back up. Once you catch back up, you can continue working each problem at your normal pace.

Furthermore, don't dwell on the problems that you were rushed on. If a problem was taking up too much time and you made a hurried guess, it must be difficult. The difficult questions are the ones you are most likely to miss anyway, so it isn't a big loss. It is better to end with more time than you need than to run out of time.

Lastly, sometimes it is beneficial to slow down if you are constantly getting ahead of time. You are always more likely to catch a careless mistake by working more slowly than quickly, and among very high-scoring test takers (those who are likely to have lots of time left over), careless errors affect the score more than mastery of material.

Secret Key #2 - Guessing is not Guesswork

You probably know that guessing is a good idea - unlike other standardized tests, there is no penalty for getting a wrong answer. Even if you have no idea about a question, you still have a 20-25% chance of getting it right.

Most test takers do not understand the impact that proper guessing can have on their score. Unless you score extremely high, guessing will significantly contribute to your final score.

Monkeys Take the Test

What most test takers don't realize is that to insure that 20-25% chance, you have to guess randomly. If you put 20 monkeys in a room to take this test, assuming they answered once per question and behaved themselves, on average they would get 20-25% of the questions correct. Put 20 test takers in the room, and the average will be much lower among guessed questions. Why?

1. The test writers intentionally writes deceptive answer choices that "look" right. A test taker has no idea about a question, so picks the "best looking" answer, which is often wrong. The monkey has no idea what looks good and what doesn't, so will consistently be lucky about 20-25% of the time.
2. Test takers will eliminate answer choices from the guessing pool based on a hunch or intuition. Simple but correct answers often get excluded, leaving a 0% chance of being correct. The monkey has no clue, and often gets lucky with the best choice.

This is why the process of elimination endorsed by most test courses is flawed and detrimental to your performance- test takers don't guess, they make an ignorant stab in the dark that is usually worse than random.

$5 Challenge

Let me introduce one of the most valuable ideas of this course- the $5 challenge:

You only mark your "best guess" if you are willing to bet $5 on it.

You only eliminate choices from guessing if you are willing to bet $5 on it.

Why $5? Five dollars is an amount of money that is small yet not insignificant, and can really add up fast (20 questions could cost you $100). Likewise, each answer choice on one question of the test will have a small impact on your overall score, but it can really add up to a lot of points in the end.

The process of elimination IS valuable. The following shows your chance of guessing it right:

If you eliminate wrong answer choices until only this many remain:	1	2	3
Chance of getting it correct:	100%	50%	33%

However, if you accidentally eliminate the right answer or go on a hunch for an incorrect answer, your chances drop dramatically: to 0%. By guessing among all the answer choices, you are GUARANTEED to have a shot at the right answer.

That's why the $5 test is so valuable- if you give up the advantage and safety of a pure guess, it had better be worth the risk.

What we still haven't covered is how to be sure that whatever guess you make is truly random. Here's the easiest way:

Always pick the first answer choice among those remaining.

Such a technique means that you have decided, **before you see a single test question**, exactly how you are going to guess- and since the order of choices tells you nothing about which one is correct, this guessing technique is perfectly random.

This section is not meant to scare you away from making educated guesses or eliminating choices- you just need to define when a choice is worth eliminating. The $5 test, along with a pre-defined random guessing strategy, is the best way to make sure you reap all of the benefits of guessing.

Secret Key #3 - Practice Smarter, Not Harder

Many test takers delay the test preparation process because they dread the awful amounts of practice time they think necessary to succeed on the test. We have refined an effective method that will take you only a fraction of the time.

There are a number of "obstacles" in your way to succeed. Among these are answering questions, finishing in time, and mastering test-taking strategies. All must be executed on the day of the test at peak performance, or your score will suffer. The test is a mental marathon that has a large impact on your future.

Just like a marathon runner, it is important to work your way up to the full challenge. So first you just worry about questions, and then time, and finally strategy:

Success Strategy

1. Find a good source for practice tests.
2. If you are willing to make a larger time investment, consider using more than one study guide- often the different approaches of multiple authors will help you "get" difficult concepts.
3. Take a practice test with no time constraints, with all study helps "open book." Take your time with questions and focus on applying strategies.
4. Take a practice test with time constraints, with all guides "open book."
5. Take a final practice test with no open material and time limits

If you have time to take more practice tests, just repeat step 5. By gradually exposing yourself to the full rigors of the test environment, you will condition your mind to the stress of test day and maximize your success.

Secret Key #4 - Prepare, Don't Procrastinate

Let me state an obvious fact: if you take the test three times, you will get three different scores. This is due to the way you feel on test day, the level of preparedness you have, and, despite the test writers' claims to the contrary, some tests WILL be easier for you than others.

Since your future depends so much on your score, you should maximize your chances of success. In order to maximize the likelihood of success, you've got to prepare in advance. This means taking practice tests and spending time learning the information and test taking strategies you will need to succeed.

Never take the test as a "practice" test, expecting that you can just take it again if you need to. Feel free to take sample tests on your own, but when you go to take the official test, be prepared, be focused, and do your best the first time!

Secret Key #5 - Test Yourself

Everyone knows that time is money. There is no need to spend too much of your time or too little of your time preparing for the test. You should only spend as much of your precious time preparing as is necessary for you to get the score you need.

Once you have taken a practice test under real conditions of time constraints, then you will know if you are ready for the test or not.

If you have scored extremely high the first time that you take the practice test, then there is not much point in spending countless hours studying. You are already there.

Benchmark your abilities by retaking practice tests and seeing how much you have improved. Once you score high enough to guarantee success, then you are ready.

If you have scored well below where you need, then knuckle down and begin studying in earnest. Check your improvement regularly through the use of practice tests under real conditions. Above all, don't worry, panic, or give up. The key is perseverance!

Then, when you go to take the test, remain confident and remember how well you did on the practice tests. If you can score high enough on a practice test, then you can do the same on the real thing.

General Strategies

The most important thing you can do is to ignore your fears and jump into the test immediately- do not be overwhelmed by any strange-sounding terms. You have to jump into the test like jumping into a pool- all at once is the easiest way.

Make Predictions

As you read and understand the question, try to guess what the answer will be. Remember that several of the answer choices are wrong, and once you begin reading them, your mind will immediately become cluttered with answer choices designed to throw you off. Your mind is typically the most focused immediately after you have read the question and digested its contents. If you can, try to predict what the correct answer will be. You may be surprised at what you can predict.

Quickly scan the choices and see if your prediction is in the listed answer choices. If it is, then you can be quite confident that you have the right answer. It still won't hurt to check the other answer choices, but most of the time, you've got it!

Answer the Question

It may seem obvious to only pick answer choices that answer the question, but the test writers can create some excellent answer choices that are wrong. Don't pick an answer just because it sounds right, or you believe it to be true. It MUST answer the question. Once you've made your selection, always go back and check it against the question and make sure that you didn't misread the question, and the answer choice does answer the question posed.

Benchmark

After you read the first answer choice, decide if you think it sounds correct or not. If it doesn't, move on to the next answer choice. If it does, mentally mark that answer choice. This doesn't mean that you've definitely selected it as your answer choice, it just means that it's the best you've seen thus far. Go ahead and read the next choice. If the next choice is worse than the one you've already selected, keep going to the next answer choice. If the next choice is better than the choice you've already selected, mentally mark the new answer choice as your best guess.

The first answer choice that you select becomes your standard. Every other answer choice must be benchmarked against that standard. That choice is correct until proven otherwise by another answer choice beating it out. Once you've decided that no other answer choice seems as good, do one final check to ensure that your answer choice answers the question posed.

Valid Information

Don't discount any of the information provided in the question. Every piece of information may be necessary to determine the correct answer. None of the information in the question is there to throw you off (while the answer choices will certainly have information to throw you off). If two seemingly unrelated topics are discussed, don't ignore either. You can be confident there is a relationship, or it wouldn't be included in the question, and you are probably going to have to determine what is that relationship to find the answer.

Avoid "Fact Traps"

Don't get distracted by a choice that is factually true. Your search is for the answer that answers the question. Stay focused and don't fall for an answer that is true but incorrect. Always go back to the question and make sure you're choosing an answer that actually answers the question and is not just a true statement. An answer can be factually correct, but it MUST answer the question asked. Additionally, two answers can both be seemingly correct, so be sure to read all of the answer choices, and make sure that you get the one that BEST answers the question.

Milk the Question

Some of the questions may throw you completely off. They might deal with a subject you have not been exposed to, or one that you haven't reviewed in years. While your lack of knowledge about the subject will be a hindrance, the question itself can give you many clues that will help you find the correct answer. Read the question carefully and look for clues. Watch particularly for adjectives and nouns describing difficult terms or words that you don't recognize. Regardless of if you completely understand a word or not, replacing it with a synonym either provided or one you more familiar with may help you to understand what the questions are asking. Rather than wracking your mind about specific detailed information concerning a difficult term or word, try to use mental substitutes that are easier to understand.

The Trap of Familiarity

Don't just choose a word because you recognize it. On difficult questions, you may not recognize a number of words in the answer choices. The test writers don't put "make-believe" words on the test; so don't think that just because you only recognize all the words in one answer choice means that answer choice must be correct. If you only recognize words in one answer choice, then focus on that one. Is it correct? Try your best to determine if it is correct. If it is, that is great, but if it doesn't, eliminate it. Each word and answer choice you eliminate increases your chances of getting the question correct, even if you then have to guess among the unfamiliar choices.

Eliminate Answers

Eliminate choices as soon as you realize they are wrong. But be careful! Make sure you consider all of the possible answer choices. Just because one appears right, doesn't mean that the next one won't be even better! The test writers will usually put more than one good answer choice for every question, so read all of them. Don't worry if you are stuck between two that seem right. By getting down to just two remaining possible choices, your odds are now 50/50. Rather than wasting too much time, play the odds. You are guessing, but guessing wisely, because you've been able to knock out some of the answer choices that you know are wrong. If you are eliminating choices and realize that the last answer choice you are left with is also obviously wrong, don't panic. Start over and consider each choice again. There may easily be something that you missed the first time and will realize on the second pass.

Tough Questions

If you are stumped on a problem or it appears too hard or too difficult, don't waste time. Move on! Remember though, if you can quickly check for obviously incorrect answer choices, your chances of guessing correctly are greatly improved. Before you completely give up, at least try to knock out a couple of possible answers. Eliminate what you can and then guess at the remaining answer choices before moving on.

Brainstorm

If you get stuck on a difficult question, spend a few seconds quickly brainstorming. Run through the complete list of possible answer choices. Look at each choice and ask yourself, "Could this answer the question satisfactorily?" Go through each answer choice and consider it independently of the other. By systematically going through all possibilities, you may find something that you would otherwise overlook. Remember that when you get stuck, it's important to try to keep moving.

Read Carefully

Understand the problem. Read the question and answer choices carefully. Don't miss the question because you misread the terms. You have plenty of time to read each question thoroughly and make sure you understand what is being asked. Yet a happy medium must be attained, so don't waste too much time. You must read carefully, but efficiently.

Face Value

When in doubt, use common sense. Always accept the situation in the problem at face value. Don't read too much into it. These problems will not require you to make huge leaps of logic. The test writers aren't trying to throw you off with a cheap trick. If you have to go beyond creativity and make a leap of logic in order to have an answer choice answer the question, then you should look at the other answer choices. Don't overcomplicate the problem by creating theoretical relationships or explanations that will warp time or space. These are normal problems rooted in reality. It's just that the applicable relationship or explanation may not be readily apparent and you have to figure things out. Use your common sense to interpret anything that isn't clear.

Prefixes

If you're having trouble with a word in the question or answer choices, try dissecting it. Take advantage of every clue that the word might include. Prefixes and suffixes can be a huge help. Usually they allow you to determine a basic meaning. Pre- means before, post- means after, pro - is positive, de- is negative. From these prefixes and suffixes, you can get an idea of the general meaning of the word and try to put it into context. Beware though of any traps. Just because con is the opposite of pro, doesn't necessarily mean congress is the opposite of progress!

Hedge Phrases

Watch out for critical "hedge" phrases, such as likely, may, can, will often, sometimes, often, almost, mostly, usually, generally, rarely, sometimes. Question writers insert these hedge phrases to cover every possibility. Often an answer choice will be wrong simply because it leaves no room for exception. Avoid answer choices that have definitive words like "exactly," and "always".

Switchback Words

Stay alert for "switchbacks". These are the words and phrases frequently used to alert you to shifts in thought. The most common switchback word is "but". Others include although, however, nevertheless, on the other hand, even though, while, in spite of, despite, regardless of.

New Information

Correct answer choices will rarely have completely new information included. Answer choices typically are straightforward reflections of the material asked about and will directly relate to the question. If a new piece of information is included in an answer choice that doesn't even seem to relate to the topic being asked about, then that answer choice is likely incorrect. All of the information needed to answer the question is usually provided for you, and so you should not have to make guesses that are unsupported or choose answer choices that require unknown information that cannot be reasoned on its own.

Time Management

On technical questions, don't get lost on the technical terms. Don't spend too much time on any one question. If you don't know what a term means, then since you don't have a dictionary, odds are you aren't going to get much further. You should immediately recognize terms as whether or not you know them. If you don't, work with the other clues that you have, the other answer choices and terms provided, but don't waste too much time trying to figure out a difficult term.

Contextual Clues

Look for contextual clues. An answer can be right but not correct. The contextual clues will help you find the answer that is most right and is correct. Understand the context in which a phrase or statement is made. This will help you make important distinctions.

Don't Panic

Panicking will not answer any questions for you. Therefore, it isn't helpful. When you first see the question, if your mind goes blank, take a deep breath. Force yourself to mechanically go through the steps of solving the problem and using the strategies you've learned.

Pace Yourself

Don't get clock fever. It's easy to be overwhelmed when you're looking at a page full of questions, your mind is full of random thoughts and feeling confused, and the clock is ticking down faster than you would like. Calm down and maintain the pace that you have set for yourself. As long as you are on track by monitoring your pace, you are guaranteed to have enough time for yourself. When you get to the last few minutes of the test, it may seem like you won't have enough time left, but if you only have as many questions as you should have left at that point, then you're right on track!

Answer Selection

The best way to pick an answer choice is to eliminate all of those that are wrong, until only one is left and confirm that is the correct answer. Sometimes though, an answer choice may immediately look right. Be careful! Take a second to make sure that the other choices are not equally obvious. Don't make a hasty mistake. There are only two times that you should stop before checking other answers. First is when you are positive that the answer choice you have selected is correct. Second is when time is almost out and you have to make a quick guess!

Check Your Work

Since you will probably not know every term listed and the answer to every question, it is important that you get credit for the ones that you do know. Don't miss any questions through careless mistakes. If at all possible, try to take a second to look back over your answer selection and make sure you've selected the correct answer choice and haven't made a costly careless mistake (such as marking an answer choice that you didn't mean to mark). This quick double check should more than pay for itself in caught mistakes for the time it costs.

Beware of Directly Quoted Answers

Sometimes an answer choice will repeat word for word a portion of the question or reference section. However, beware of such exact duplication – it may be a trap! More than likely, the correct choice will paraphrase or summarize a point, rather than being exactly the same wording.

Slang

Scientific sounding answers are better than slang ones. An answer choice that begins "To compare the outcomes…" is much more likely to be correct than one that begins "Because some people insisted…"

Extreme Statements

Avoid wild answers that throw out highly controversial ideas that are proclaimed as established fact. An answer choice that states the "process should be used in certain situations, if…" is much more likely to be correct than one that states the "process should be discontinued completely." The first is a calm rational statement and doesn't even make a definitive, uncompromising stance, using a hedge word "if" to provide wiggle room, whereas the second choice is a radical idea and far more extreme.

Answer Choice Families

When you have two or more answer choices that are direct opposites or parallels, one of them is usually the correct answer. For instance, if one answer choice states "x increases" and another answer choice states "x decreases" or "y increases," then those two or three answer choices are very similar in construction and fall into the same family of answer choices. A family of answer choices is when two or three answer choices are very similar in construction, and yet often have a directly opposite meaning. Usually the correct answer choice will be in that family of answer choices. The "odd man out" or answer choice that doesn't seem to fit the parallel construction of the other answer choices is more likely to be incorrect.

Special Report: How to Overcome Test Anxiety

The very nature of tests caters to some level of anxiety, nervousness or tension, just as we feel for any important event that occurs in our lives. A little bit of anxiety or nervousness can be a good thing. It helps us with motivation, and makes achievement just that much sweeter. However, too much anxiety can be a problem; especially if it hinders our ability to function and perform.

"Test anxiety," is the term that refers to the emotional reactions that some test-takers experience when faced with a test or exam. Having a fear of testing and exams is based upon a rational fear, since the test-taker's performance can shape the course of an academic career. Nevertheless, experiencing excessive fear of examinations will only interfere with the test-takers ability to perform, and his/her chances to be successful.

There are a large variety of causes that can contribute to the development and sensation of test anxiety. These include, but are not limited to lack of performance and worrying about issues surrounding the test.

Lack of Preparation

Lack of preparation can be identified by the following behaviors or situations:

Not scheduling enough time to study, and therefore cramming the night before the test or exam

Managing time poorly, to create the sensation that there is not enough time to do everything

Failing to organize the text information in advance, so that the study material consists of the entire text and not simply the pertinent information
Poor overall studying habits

Worrying, on the other hand, can be related to both the test taker, or many other factors around him/her that will be affected by the results of the test. These include worrying about:

Previous performances on similar exams, or exams in general
How friends and other students are achieving
The negative consequences that will result from a poor grade or failure

There are three primary elements to test anxiety. Physical components, which involve the same typical bodily reactions as those to acute anxiety (to be discussed below). Emotional factors have to do with fear or panic. Mental or cognitive issues concerning attention spans and memory abilities.

Physical Signals

There are many different symptoms of test anxiety, and these are not limited to mental and emotional strain. Frequently there are a range of physical signals that will let a test taker know that he/she is suffering from test anxiety. These bodily changes can include the following:

Perspiring
Sweaty palms
Wet, trembling hands
Nausea
Dry mouth

A knot in the stomach

Headache

Faintness

Muscle tension

Aching shoulders, back and neck

Rapid heart beat

Feeling too hot/cold

To recognize the sensation of test anxiety, a test-taker should monitor him/herself for the following sensations:

The physical distress symptoms as listed above
Emotional sensitivity, expressing emotional feelings such as the need to cry or laugh too much, or a sensation of anger or helplessness
A decreased ability to think, causing the test-taker to blank out or have racing thoughts that are hard to organize or control.

Though most students will feel some level of anxiety when faced with a test or exam, the majority can cope with that anxiety and maintain it at a manageable level. However, those who cannot are faced with a very real and very serious condition, which can and should be controlled for the immeasurable benefit of this sufferer.

Naturally, these sensations lead to negative results for the testing experience. The most common effects of test anxiety have to do with nervousness and mental blocking.

Nervousness

Nervousness can appear in several different levels:

The test-taker's difficulty, or even inability to read and understand the questions on the test
The difficulty or inability to organize thoughts to a coherent form
The difficulty or inability to recall key words and concepts relating to the testing questions (especially essays)
The receipt of poor grades on a test, though the test material was well known by the test taker

Conversely, a person may also experience mental blocking, which involves:

Blanking out on test questions
Only remembering the correct answers to the questions when the test has already finished.

Fortunately for test anxiety sufferers, beating these feelings, to a large degree, has to do with proper preparation. When a test taker has a feeling of preparedness, then anxiety will be dramatically lessened.

The first step to resolving anxiety issues is to distinguish which of the two types of anxiety are being suffered. If the anxiety is a direct result of a lack of preparation, this should be considered a normal reaction, and the anxiety level (as opposed to the test results) shouldn't be anything to worry about. However, if, when adequately prepared, the test-taker still panics, blanks out, or seems to overreact, this is not a fully rational reaction. While this can be considered normal too, there are many ways to combat and overcome these effects.

Remember that anxiety cannot be entirely eliminated, however, there are ways to minimize it, to make the anxiety easier to manage. Preparation is one of the best ways to minimize test anxiety. Therefore the following techniques are wise in order to best fight off any anxiety that may want to build.

To begin with, try to avoid cramming before a test, whenever it is possible. By trying to memorize an entire term's worth of information in one day, you'll be shocking your system, and not giving yourself a very good chance to absorb the information. This is an easy path to anxiety, so for those who suffer from test anxiety, cramming should not even be considered an option.

Instead of cramming, work throughout the semester to combine all of the material which is presented throughout the semester, and work on it gradually as the course goes by, making sure to master the main concepts first, leaving minor details for a week or so before the test.

To study for the upcoming exam, be sure to pose questions that may be on the examination, to gauge the ability to answer them by integrating the ideas from your texts, notes and lectures, as well as any supplementary readings.

If it is truly impossible to cover all of the information that was covered in that particular term, concentrate on the most important portions, that can be covered very well. Learn these concepts as best as possible, so that when the test comes, a goal can be made to use these concepts as presentations of your knowledge.

In addition to study habits, changes in attitude are critical to beating a struggle with test anxiety. In fact, an improvement of the perspective over the entire test-taking experience can actually help a test taker to enjoy studying and therefore improve the overall experience. Be certain not to overemphasize the significance of the grade - know that the result of the test is neither a reflection of self worth, nor is it a measure of intelligence; one grade will not predict a person's future success.

To improve an overall testing outlook, the following steps should be tried:

Keeping in mind that the most reasonable expectation for taking a test is to expect to try to demonstrate as much of what you know as you possibly can.
Reminding ourselves that a test is only one test; this is not the only one, and there will be others.
The thought of thinking of oneself in an irrational, all-or-nothing term should be avoided at all costs.
A reward should be designated for after the test, so there's something to look forward to. Whether it be going to a movie, going out to eat, or simply visiting friends, schedule it in advance, and do it no matter what result is expected on the exam.

Test-takers should also keep in mind that the basics are some of the most important things, even beyond anti-anxiety techniques and studying. Never neglect the basic social, emotional and biological needs, in order to try to absorb information. In order to best achieve, these three factors must be held as just as important as the studying itself.

Study Steps

Remember the following important steps for studying:

Maintain healthy nutrition and exercise habits. Continue both your recreational activities and social pass times. These both contribute to your physical and emotional well being.

Be certain to get a good amount of sleep, especially the night before the test, because when you're overtired you are not able to perform to the best of your best ability.
Keep the studying pace to a moderate level by taking breaks when they are needed, and varying the work whenever possible, to keep the mind fresh instead of getting bored.
When enough studying has been done that all the material that can be learned has been learned, and the test taker is prepared for the test, stop studying and do something relaxing such as listening to music, watching a movie, or taking a warm bubble bath.

There are also many other techniques to minimize the uneasiness or apprehension that is experienced along with test anxiety before, during, or even after the examination. In fact, there are a great deal of things that can be done to stop anxiety from interfering with lifestyle and performance. Again, remember that anxiety will not be eliminated entirely, and it shouldn't be. Otherwise that "up" feeling for exams would not exist, and most of us depend on that sensation to perform better than usual. However, this anxiety has to be at a level that is manageable.

Of course, as we have just discussed, being prepared for the exam is half the battle right away. Attending all classes, finding out what knowledge will be expected on the exam, and knowing the exam schedules are easy steps to lowering anxiety. Keeping up with work will remove the need to cram, and efficient study habits will eliminate wasted time. Studying should be done in an ideal location for concentration, so that it is simple to become interested in the material and give it complete attention. A method such as SQ3R (Survey, Question, Read, Recite, Review) is a wonderful key to follow to make sure that the study habits are as effective as possible, especially in the case of learning from a textbook. Flashcards are great techniques for memorization. Learning to take good notes will mean that notes will be full of useful information, so that less sifting will need to be done to seek out what is pertinent for studying. Reviewing notes after class and then again on occasion will keep the information fresh in the mind. From notes that have been taken summary sheets and outlines can be made for simpler reviewing.

A study group can also be a very motivational and helpful place to study, as there will be a sharing of ideas, all of the minds can work together, to make sure that everyone understands, and the studying will be made more interesting because it will be a social occasion.

Basically, though, as long as the test-taker remains organized and self confident, with efficient study habits, less time will need to be spent studying, and higher grades will be achieved.

To become self confident, there are many useful steps. The first of these is "self talk." It has been shown through extensive research, that self-talk for students who suffer from test anxiety, should be well monitored, in order to make sure that it contributes to self confidence as opposed to sinking the student. Frequently the self talk of test-anxious students is negative or self-defeating, thinking that everyone else is smarter and faster, that they always mess up, and that if they don't do well, they'll fail the entire course. It is important to decreasing anxiety that awareness is made of self talk. Try writing any negative self thoughts and then disputing them with a positive statement instead. Begin self-encouragement as though it was a friend speaking. Repeat positive statements to help reprogram the mind to believing in successes instead of failures.

Helpful Techniques

Other extremely helpful techniques include:

Self-visualization of doing well and reaching goals
While aiming for an "A" level of understanding, don't try to "overprotect" by setting your expectations lower. This will only convince the mind to stop studying in order to meet the lower expectations.
Don't make comparisons with the results or habits of other students. These are individual factors, and different things work for different people, causing different results.
Strive to become an expert in learning what works well, and what can be done in order to improve. Consider collecting this data in a journal.
Create rewards for after studying instead of doing things before studying that will only turn into avoidance behaviors.
Make a practice of relaxing - by using methods such as progressive relaxation, self-hypnosis, guided imagery, etc - in order to make relaxation an automatic sensation.
Work on creating a state of relaxed concentration so that concentrating will take on the focus of the mind, so that none will be wasted on worrying.
Take good care of the physical self by eating well and getting enough sleep.
Plan in time for exercise and stick to this plan.

Beyond these techniques, there are other methods to be used before, during and after the test that will help the test-taker perform well in addition to overcoming anxiety.

Before the exam comes the academic preparation. This involves establishing a study schedule and beginning at least one week before the actual date of the test. By doing this, the anxiety of not having enough time to study for the test will be automatically eliminated. Moreover, this will make the studying a much more effective experience, ensuring that the learning will be an easier process. This relieves much undue pressure on the test-taker.

Summary sheets, note cards, and flash cards with the main concepts and examples of these main concepts should be prepared in advance of the actual studying time. A topic should never be eliminated from this process. By omitting a topic because it isn't expected to be on the test is only setting up the test-taker for anxiety should it actually appear on the exam. Utilize the course syllabus for laying out the topics that should be studied. Carefully go over the notes that were made in class, paying special attention to any of the issues that the professor took special care to emphasize while lecturing in class. In the textbooks, use the chapter review, or if possible, the chapter tests, to begin your review.

It may even be possible to ask the instructor what information will be covered on the exam, or what the format of the exam will be (for example, multiple choice, essay, free form, true-false). Additionally, see if it is possible to find out how many questions will be on the test. If a review sheet or sample test has been offered by the professor, make good use of it, above anything else, for the preparation for the test. Another great resource for getting to know the examination is reviewing tests from previous semesters. Use these tests to review, and aim to achieve a 100% score on each of the possible topics. With a few exceptions, the goal that you set for yourself is the highest one that you will reach.

Take all of the questions that were assigned as homework, and rework them to any other possible course material. The more problems reworked, the more skill and confidence will form as a result. When forming the solution to a problem, write out each of the steps. Don't simply do head work. By doing as many steps on paper as possible, much clarification and therefore confidence will be formed. Do this with as many homework problems as possible, before checking the answers. By checking the answer after each problem, a reinforcement will exist, that will not be on the exam. Study situations should be as exam-like as possible, to prime the test-taker's system for the experience. By waiting to check the answers at the end, a psychological advantage will be formed, to decrease the stress factor.

Another fantastic reason for not cramming is the avoidance of confusion in concepts, especially when it comes to mathematics. 8-10 hours of study will become one hundred percent more effective if it is spread out over a week or at least several days, instead of doing it all in one sitting. Recognize that the human brain requires time in order to assimilate new material, so frequent breaks and a span of study time over several days will be much more beneficial.

Additionally, don't study right up until the point of the exam. Studying should stop a minimum of one hour before the exam begins. This allows the brain to rest and put things in their proper order. This will also provide the time to become as relaxed as possible when going into the examination room. The test-taker will also have time to eat well and eat sensibly. Know that the brain needs food as much as the rest of the body. With enough food and enough sleep, as well as a relaxed attitude, the body and the mind are primed for success.

Avoid any anxious classmates who are talking about the exam. These students only spread anxiety, and are not worth sharing the anxious sentimentalities.

Before the test also involves creating a positive attitude, so mental preparation should also be a point of concentration. There are many keys to creating a positive attitude. Should fears become rushing in, make a visualization of taking the exam, doing well, and seeing an A written on the paper. Write out a list of affirmations that will bring a feeling of confidence, such as "I am doing well in my English class," "I studied well and know my material," "I enjoy this class." Even if the affirmations aren't believed at first, it sends a positive message to the subconscious which will result in an alteration of the overall belief system, which is the system that creates reality.

If a sensation of panic begins, work with the fear and imagine the very worst! Work through the entire scenario of not passing the test, failing the entire course, and dropping out of school, followed by not getting a job, and pushing a shopping cart through the dark alley where you'll live. This will place things into perspective! Then, practice deep breathing and create a visualization of the opposite situation - achieving an "A" on the exam, passing the entire course, receiving the degree at a graduation ceremony.

On the day of the test, there are many things to be done to ensure the best results, as well as the most calm outlook. The following stages are suggested in order to maximize test-taking potential:

Begin the examination day with a moderate breakfast, and avoid any coffee or beverages with caffeine if the test taker is prone to jitters. Even people who are used to managing caffeine can feel jittery or light-headed when it is taken on a test day.
Attempt to do something that is relaxing before the examination begins. As last minute cramming clouds the mastering of overall concepts, it is better to use this time to create a calming outlook.
Be certain to arrive at the test location well in advance, in order to provide time to select a location that is away from doors, windows and other distractions, as well as giving enough time to relax before the test begins.
Keep away from anxiety generating classmates who will upset the sensation of stability and relaxation that is being attempted before the exam.

Should the waiting period before the exam begins cause anxiety, create a self-distraction by reading a light magazine or something else that is relaxing and simple.

During the exam itself, read the entire exam from beginning to end, and find out how much time should be allotted to each individual problem. Once writing the exam, should more time be taken for a problem, it should be abandoned, in order to begin another problem. If there is time at the end, the unfinished problem can always be returned to and completed.

Read the instructions very carefully - twice - so that unpleasant surprises won't follow during or after the exam has ended.

When writing the exam, pretend that the situation is actually simply the completion of homework within a library, or at home. This will assist in forming a relaxed atmosphere, and will allow the brain extra focus for the complex thinking function.

Begin the exam with all of the questions with which the most confidence is felt. This will build the confidence level regarding the entire exam and will begin a quality momentum. This will also create encouragement for trying the problems where uncertainty resides.

Going with the "gut instinct" is always the way to go when solving a problem. Second guessing should be avoided at all costs. Have confidence in the ability to do well.

For essay questions, create an outline in advance that will keep the mind organized and make certain that all of the points are remembered. For multiple choice, read every answer, even if the correct one has been spotted - a better one may exist.

Continue at a pace that is reasonable and not rushed, in order to be able to work carefully. Provide enough time to go over the answers at the end, to check for small errors that can be corrected.

Should a feeling of panic begin, breathe deeply, and think of the feeling of the body releasing sand through its pores. Visualize a calm, peaceful place, and include all of the sights, sounds and sensations of this image. Continue the deep breathing, and take a few minutes to continue this with closed eyes. When all is well again, return to the test.

If a "blanking" occurs for a certain question, skip it and move on to the next question. There will be time to return to the other question later. Get everything done that can be done, first, to guarantee all the grades that can be compiled, and to build all of the confidence possible. Then return to the weaker questions to build the marks from there.

Remember, one's own reality can be created, so as long as the belief is there, success will follow. And remember: anxiety can happen later, right now, there's an exam to be written!

After the examination is complete, whether there is a feeling for a good grade or a bad grade, don't dwell on the exam, and be certain to follow through on the reward that was promised...and enjoy it! Don't dwell on any mistakes that have been made, as there is nothing that can be done at this point anyway.

Additionally, don't begin to study for the next test right away. Do something relaxing for a while, and let the mind relax and prepare itself to begin absorbing information again.

From the results of the exam - both the grade and the entire experience, be certain to learn from what has gone on. Perfect studying habits and work some more on confidence in order to make the next examination experience even better than the last one.

Learn to avoid places where openings occurred for laziness, procrastination and day dreaming.

Use the time between this exam and the next one to better learn to relax, even learning to relax on cue, so that any anxiety can be controlled during the next exam. Learn how to relax the body. Slouch in your chair if that helps. Tighten and then relax all of the different muscle groups, one group at a time, beginning with the feet and then working all the way up to the neck and face. This will ultimately relax the muscles more than they were to begin with. Learn how to breathe deeply and comfortably, and focus on this breathing going in and out as a relaxing thought. With every exhale, repeat the word "relax."

As common as test anxiety is, it is very possible to overcome it. Make yourself one of the test-takers who overcome this frustrating hindrance.

Special Report: Retaking the Test: What Are Your Chances at Improving Your Score?

After going through the experience of taking a major test, many test takers feel that once is enough. The test usually comes during a period of transition in the test taker's life, and taking the test is only one of a series of important events. With so many distractions and conflicting recommendations, it may be difficult for a test taker to rationally determine whether or not he should retake the test after viewing his scores.

The importance of the test usually only adds to the burden of the retake decision. However, don't be swayed by emotion. There a few simple questions that you can ask yourself to guide you as you try to determine whether a retake would improve your score:

1. What went wrong? Why wasn't your score what you expected?

Can you point to a single factor or problem that you feel caused the low score? Were you sick on test day? Was there an emotional upheaval in your life that caused a distraction? Were you late for the test or not able to use the full time allotment? If you can point to any of these specific, individual problems, then a retake should definitely be considered.

2. Is there enough time to improve?

Many problems that may show up in your score report may take a lot of time for improvement. A deficiency in a particular math skill may require weeks or months of tutoring and studying to improve. If you have enough time to improve an identified weakness, then a retake should definitely be considered.

3. How will additional scores be used? Will a score average, highest score, or most recent score be used?

Different test scores may be handled completely differently. If you've taken the test multiple times, sometimes your highest score is used, sometimes your average score is computed and used, and sometimes your most recent score is used. Make sure you understand what method will be used to evaluate your scores, and use that to help you determine whether a retake should be considered.

4. Are my practice test scores significantly higher than my actual test score?

If you have taken a lot of practice tests and are consistently scoring at a much higher level than your actual test score, then you should consider a retake. However, if you've taken five practice tests and only one of your scores was higher than your actual test score, or if your practice test scores were only slightly higher than your actual test score, then it is unlikely that you will significantly increase your score.

5. Do I need perfect scores or will I be able to live with this score? Will this score still allow me to follow my dreams?

What kind of score is acceptable to you? Is your current score "good enough?" Do you have to have a certain score in order to pursue the future of your dreams? If you won't be happy with your current score, and there's no way that you could live with it, then you should consider a retake. However, don't get your hopes up. If you are looking for significant improvement, that may or may not be possible. But if you won't be happy otherwise, it is at least worth the effort.

Remember that there are other considerations. To achieve your dream, it is likely that your grades may also be taken into account. A great test score is usually not the only thing necessary to succeed. Make sure that you aren't overemphasizing the importance of a high test score.

Furthermore, a retake does not always result in a higher score. Some test takers will score lower on a retake, rather than higher. One study shows that one-fourth of test takers will achieve a significant improvement in test score, while one-sixth of test takers will actually show a decrease. While this shows that most test takers will improve, the majority will only improve their scores a little and a retake may not be worth the test taker's effort.

Finally, if a test is taken only once and is considered in the added context of good grades on the part of a test taker, the person reviewing the grades and scores may be tempted to assume that the test taker just had a bad day while taking the test, and may discount the low test score in favor of the high grades. But if the test is retaken and the scores are approximately the same, then the validity of the low scores are only confirmed. Therefore, a retake could actually hurt a test taker by definitely bracketing a test taker's score ability to a limited range.

Special Report: Additional Bonus Material

Due to our efforts to try to keep this book to a manageable length, we've created a link that will give you access to all of your additional bonus material.

Please visit http://www.mometrix.com/bonus948/orthopaedic to access the information.